# MISSION POSSIBLE

By L. Marlene Payne, M.D.

**ISBN-13: 978-1507536230**

**ISBN-10: 1507536232**

# DEDICATION

I would like to dedicate this book to two wonderful men in my life:
my husband John and my son J.D. Payne

# Table of Contents

# ACKNOWLEDGEMENTS

I am deeply indebted to my family for their help and support for this book. My husband John Payne, my siblings Barbara Mellen, Carol Morgan, Dan Jones, and Ken Jones, and my children Jenny Dundee, J.D. Payne, and Heather Petersen read and commented on the chapters. My son J.D. Payne and my nephew Vance Mellen were enormously helpful and patient in getting the book ready for publication.

I am grateful to all those who contributed their thoughts and experiences for the last several chapters. I am also thankful for the missionaries who faithfully came to their sessions and taught me so much about the challenges and joys of missionary work.

# Introduction

*So how do you best respond when mental or emotional challenges confront you or those you love?... If things continue to be debilitating, seek the advice of reputable people with certified training, professional skills, and good values. Be honest with them about your history and your struggles. Prayerfully and responsibly consider the counsel they give and the solutions they prescribe. If you had appendicitis, God would expect you to seek a priesthood blessing and get the best medical care available. So too with emotional disorders. Our Father in Heaven expects us to use all of the marvelous gifts He has provided in this glorious dispensation.*[i]

--Elder Jeffrey R. Holland

Elder White* rose to say goodbye. He was the last missionary I treated at the end of forty years as a psychiatrist. He gave me a firm parting handshake, and I watched him go down the stairs wondering how he would apply all he had learned on his mission. He had learned that he was bipolar. He was on three medications to keep his mood steady after months of patient trial and error to find the right combination and dosage. He had learned that he had attention deficit hyperactivity disorder and couldn't tolerate any of the ADHD medications because they destabilized his mood, so he also learned behavioral skills for executive functioning (the mental skills coordinated by the frontal lobe such as planning, managing time, and remembering details). He had learned to work with exceedingly difficult companions, the kind that get transferred every six weeks because they are so hard to be with, and he had remained with them for two or three transfers. In doing that, he had learned that his

*All names of patients have been changed.

childhood under the hand of an angry, unempathetic, blaming parent had prepared him to work with difficult people, and had given him a gentleness with the rough ones. He learned to dismantle the shell he had built around himself so that he could communicate with others and show his real self. He learned that he could grapple with a challenge and come away the victor.

I had such admiration for the courage of the missionaries I helped. They chose to stay on their missions even though they were suffering. Missionaries were referred to me for help with depression, bipolar disorder, anxiety disorders, obsessive-compulsive disorder, attention deficit hyperactivity disorder, autism (Asperger's syndrome), and other conditions. Some knew they had these disorders when they came, but often I was the first doctor to diagnose their problems. Sometimes I would work with a dozen missionaries at a time in my practice, sometimes only with one or two, but they were a constant presence throughout my years of service. I would see them once a week in the beginning to take their history, make a diagnosis, and start treatment. When they were feeling better I would see them every other week for a few times, then cut back to once a month. We used the fifty minute sessions to discuss their past, present, and future and to adjust their medications as needed. I felt it was vital that we continue meeting for the duration of their mission so they would feel a connection with me, and so I could know them well. That way I was able to give them support when they had difficulties. This was particularly important in helping them to stay on their missions.

When Elder Holland gave his talk in October, 2013, I was amazed. When I first began my career as a psychiatrist forty years ago, there was an attitude in general society as well as in the Church of Jesus Christ of Latter-day Saints that mental illness represented a personal failure, that it was optional or even shameful.

A friend named Louise Degn recognized this problem and made a documentary film in the early 1970's about depression for members of the church. In her film she stressed that depression was not a weakness of character but a medical illness which required medical care and therapy. It did not help to tell depressed people that they needed to stop thinking so much about themselves and go out to serve someone else so they could feel better. It seems obvious to us now, but it was revolutionary forty years ago. Many surrounding stakes invited me to talk as they showed the film to their members. People were so grateful for that message.

Notwithstanding the progress in attitudes toward mental illness, the talk by Elder Holland was astounding because he acknowledged that he had been depressed as a young man, and that depression is a medical illness. He recommended that people should seek medical help for it and other mental illnesses. This should include the use of medicine when prescribed by "reputable people with certified training, professional skills, and good values." This counsel was given in General Conference in a talk heard around the world.

Factors that have helped change the public perception of mental illness include the expanding scientific base of information about neuroanatomy and neurophysiology. There has been much progress in knowledge of neurochemistry and its role in mental illness. The following list illustrates some of the clinical advances:

- Development of many new medications providing a far more effective array of tools to treat mental disorders
- Optimal brain nutrition like omega three fatty acids, vitamin D3, B vitamins, and SAM-E
- Deep brain stimulation for treatment of depression
- Cognitive behavioral therapy for OCD, anxiety disorders, and depression
- Mentalization training for character disorders like borderline personality disorder
- Bright light therapy for seasonal affective disorders and sleep disorders
- Treatment for sleep disorders diagnosed in a sleep laboratory (ex: sleep apnea, narcolepsy, periodic limb movement disorder) Treatment can be accomplished with a CPAP mask or a mandibular repositioning device.

In addition to these clinical advances is the exciting new information derived from genetic testing. Genetic testing has so much potential to help suffering people. The tests can assess:

- Genetic vulnerabilities for psychiatric disorders
- Genetic ability to respond to various psychiatric medications
- Rapid metabolizers who break down medications too quickly to achieve adequate therapeutic blood levels

- Slow metabolizers who break down medications too slowly, build up a high blood level, and develop many side effects
- Those who have a genetic variation of the MTHFR gene (almost 50% of the population). This gene regulates an enzyme that contributes a methyl group to the B vitamin called folate. Folate then donates this methyl group in the synthesis of major neurotransmitters like dopamine, serotonin, and norepinephrine. If a person has this genetic inability to attach a methyl group on folate, they have low levels of these major neurotransmitters. They consequently do not respond well to medications like antidepressants for depression or stimulants for ADHD. Recently substances (e.g. Deplin) have become available to supply methylated folate and fill in the gap in synthesis.

Underlying all these treatment options is the therapeutic alliance, the foundation of psychiatric treatment. This bond is forged as the patient and therapist work together to restore well being. It is based on mutual trust and respect. The therapist helps the patient put feelings into words and find better ways to communicate and resolve these feelings. Patients learn to nurture their own and others' needs. They learn to find joy in creativity, service, and spiritual growth. Let me give a few examples of how this communication helps.

I worked with a sister missionary who was suffering from depression. We treated it, and she was much better, but her companion's mother died unexpectedly. The companion went home abruptly for five days, leaving my patient on her own to find members of the ward to stay with her, arrange rides, and do all their work by herself. Under this increased stress, she slid back into depression. When she came to her next session in despair, I reminded her that stress causes depression through elevated cortisol levels which have a negative impact on brain chemistry. This sister and I had a strong bond, and she felt calmer as I reassured her that we would get her back on track. I also temporarily increased her antidepressant, and she responded well.

An elder came for treatment of depression, and as we talked I learned that his father, who lived in another country and who was a member of the stake presidency, was still relying on his son to do the accounting for the father's business even while he was on his mission. I contacted our mission president and explained the situation. He called the elder's stake president who told the father not to expect his son to be an accountant while on his mission. Without that added responsibility, my patient felt much better.

Another elder from a small farming town in Utah and a close, loving family was intractably homesick. When the summer approached, all he could think about was that his father and brothers would be riding horses into the mountains for a week of camping, hiking, and fishing. I asked the mission president if this elder could call his mother when his homesickness became overwhelming, and the president agreed as long as the elder asked his permission each time he needed to call. The elder did not abuse the privilege but felt much better knowing he could call when he needed to. It helped that I shared his love of horses, mountains, and hiking.

Another elder yawned his way through our sessions. I wondered if he were bored, often a sign in therapy that patients were working at a superficial level and avoiding underlying problems. He assured me that he was always this way, chronically exhausted. This could be a symptom of depression, but he wasn't depressed. I checked his hematocrit for anemia and his thyroid hormone levels for hypothyroidism, but they were normal. I thought he probably had a sleep disorder, perhaps sleep apnea, which would require a sleep study to make the diagnosis. This was not possible on a mission and would have to wait until he returned home. In the interim. I called his mission president, explained his problem, and asked if the elder could sleep on extra half an hour in the morning and take a nap at lunch. The mission president graciously agreed. The yawning almost disappeared.

Other missionaries required much more complicated and intense treatment, and most of them chose to stay so they could finish their missions. The mission exposed their vulnerabilities but also gave them opportunity to grow.

Many came for help at the beginning of their missions, so I was able to see their progress not only emotionally and psychologically, but spiritually as well. I learned that missionaries grew in many ways. They thought less about themselves and more about their investigators as time went on. They developed a love and empathy for those they taught. They deepened their ability to communicate and work through problems with their companions. They learned the immense value of bending their will to fit the yoke of obedience. They could see in the lives of their investigators that while we all have our free agency there are consequences to our choices. Most of them learned to rely on the Lord and receive counsel and direction from the Holy Ghost. They developed deeper testimonies, stronger faith, and often more humility.

As I saw their growth I began to understand how important it was for them to stay for their whole mission. If they left early, it truncated that growth. They could of course continue to progress spiritually even if they went home early, but the growth was slower. I watched my son, John Daniel, develop spiritually on his mission in ways that took me at least fifteen years to reach without a mission.

My son had an experience that helped our family see the tender mercies that the Lord extends to His missionaries. J.D. served in the Rome, Italy mission and prayed throughout that he could help to bring a family into the Church. Twice he and his companion had taught a family who accepted the Gospel and agreed to be baptized.

Each time, as they were filling the baptismal font, the family contacted them and said that they had changed their minds and wanted nothing further to do with the Church.

We went to Rome to pick up J.D. at the end of his mission. He came down to Rome from Pescara by bus, and on the bus he met a man who became interested in the Church. Since J.D. was leaving, he passed his name to the elders who took his place.

The following year my son asked if he could return to Rome over spring break. Excited to see the members and some old investigators, he went to his last city first. When he arrived in Church on Sunday, they announced the confirmation of a family that had been baptized the previous evening. As they put their hands on the father's head, JD realized that he knew the man. It was the man he had invited, the last invite of his entire mission, being confirmed a member of the Church--and his entire family with him. After the meeting JD walked up to him. The man looked at him a moment, and then his face lit up. "You!" he said with a surprised joyfulness. "You!" JD said back to him, equally surprised, equally joyful. "Thank you," the man whispered, as they embraced. "No, thank *you*," JD returned. "I looked for you my entire mission."

As I began to understand the spiritual importance of missions, I developed a desire to help missionaries finish their service. That meant I needed to help them through their difficulties, to help them be comfortable and stable, and to get back to their best selves. Then they could endure the stresses and hard work so that they could fulfill the opportunities for growth and joy that are to be found in missions.

I have written this book to share information about psychiatric conditions which may have been unknown to missionaries, their families, or their leaders. It is important to know that most psychiatric conditions are treatable, and those who suffer with these problems can usually finish their missions. The following chapters share a few of my patients' stories and are organized under the heading of the diagnosis I was treating. Although I saw many missionaries in each diagnostic category, each was unique. I learned that there was a need for many different kinds of personalities to reach many different kinds of people. There was no ideal missionary. They were all important and they all deserved the opportunity to grow and enjoy their missions.

## Chapter 1: Bipolar Disorder

*Manic thought initially gallops along in a straight line but chaos ensues as the mania progresses.*

*Custance's thoughts took flight with his mood. "As I sit here looking out of the windows of the ward," he wrote, "I see flocks of seagulls who have been driven inland by the extreme cold. The mere sight of these seagulls sets up immediately and virtually simultaneously in my mind the following trains of thoughts:*

1. A pond called Seagulls' Spring near my home.
2. *Mermaids, i.e. "Sea girls," sirens, Lorelei, Mother Seager's syrup, syrup of figs, the blasted fig-tree in the Gospels, Professor Joad who could not accept Jesus as the supremely perfect Man owing to particular incident...*
3. *Gulls equal girls, lovely girls, lovelies, film-stars, countless stars in the infinite wastes of space, query: is space really infinite? According to Einstein it is not...*

from *Exuberance* by Kay Redfield Jamison[ii]

Elder Christian Schuff was a marvel to me. When we met he had been on his mission for fourteen months with ten months to go. He was struggling with depression. As his story unfolded, I thought, "Anyone would be depressed with this history. He is here on this mission by the tender mercy of the Lord."

He had been raised in a Mennonite community in a foreign country. The sect his family belonged to was very strict, negative, and critical. The preacher was a "hellfire and damnation" sort. They spoke German, and he was educated in German with no exposure to

English. He remembered a teacher in elementary school who whipped him for not properly following the lesson. There was a prolonged drought in their country, causing his father's business to fail and forcing the family to move to another country when he was ten years old. The poverty in his family was hard on his father, a nice man sometimes, but one who could have a real temper. They were in debt, the father was under great stress, and he was very hard on Christian. The family picked strawberries to make ends meet. His brother was faster than he was, bringing his father's wrath upon him. His mother also had a strong temper and would use a whip on the bottom to discipline them, so he felt no support at home.

School was no better. The family remained Mennonite but lived in the larger community of English speaking people. He was sent to a regular middle school and struggled to learn in a language he could not understand. He wore overalls or second hand clothes to school, spoke only a few words of English with a German accent, and was clearly very different. The other students were abusive to him on the playground and school bus, and no adult intervened to protect him. He thought the others were mean because there was something wrong with him. He became depressed and thought, "What is the purpose of this life when it is so hard to live?"

When Christian was fourteen years old, his parents took him out of school, and he began to work full time. He felt that his life was at a standstill, he was not learning anything, and he had no future to look forward to. He said, "When I was eighteen I began to realize that there was something missing. I often thought life pointless to live without knowing the purpose of it; I felt emptiness. There was a desire within me to know why I existed. I began to seek answers by reading books. In the books I read, I found a way to overcome depression, but it was not happiness. Reading these books made me realize how much there is to life, yet the purpose of it all still seemed to be missing. It seemed to me that every man had his own image of

God, rather than seeking to know who God really is. I knew that the explanation to our existence had to be out there."

When he was twenty years old, he finally realized that the true answers would have to come from God. Christian prayed that he might find the truth. Two weeks later he passed a sign that said, "I am the Way, the Truth, and the Life." He googled "Jesus Christ" and had a distinct impression that the first link was the best. It was the Church of Jesus Christ of Latter Day Saints website. He read about the Book of Mormon and that it was another testament of Jesus Christ. It was free, so he ordered it, and it was delivered by two missionaries who also taught him the first discussion. They left a pamphlet about Joseph Smith, and as he read it that night he felt the Spirit for the first time. Christian became very excited that God still speaks to His prophets. As he pondered what he was learning, he felt the Spirit many times and knew the Gospel was true. He received the remaining discussions and was asked if he would like to be baptized. He wanted to wait until he turned twenty-one out of respect for his family.

Christian said, "I felt awful for hurting my family, but every time I prayed about joining the Church I had the same feeling; if I did not join the Church then I would remain in the same dark and confusing world I had always known. It was the hardest time of my life, seeing my family hurting because of me." After Christian turned twenty-one, he did get baptized, much to the distress of his family. They suggested that he move out, but he wanted to show them that he still loved them and that the Church of Jesus Christ would not stand between them. After a few weeks, they realized that he was still their son. They relaxed and began to enjoy one another's company again.

Soon after his baptism he came on his mission. His trainer was just like the kids in middle school. He was very good at belittling people and did it as often as possible. He ridiculed Elder Schuff to their roommates and made fun of the way he taught. Fortunately he was with that companion for only one transfer, and then went on to his breaker. This companion was pleasant but really into sports, and they did not connect. As his mission unfolded, it was apparent that his earlier life experiences were taking a toll on him. He was insecure and anxious, especially in large meetings, and dreaded criticism. He especially felt uncomfortable around "prideful, competitive, and intellectual" people. He began to get depressed again.

When Elder Schuff came to see me, he had symptoms of sleep impairment (multiple awakenings all through the night with dreams in which he was helpless, powerless, terrified), loss of appetite, fatigue, cognitive impairment (including problems with concentration and memory), lack of enjoyment in life, hopelessness, sadness, anxiety, irritability, lack of motivation, a wish to remain in his room rather than interacting with people, critical thoughts about himself, and loss of the ability to feel the Holy Ghost. He had all the symptoms of depression except feeling suicidal.

Elder Schuff had a kind face and a beautiful smile. It was surprising to note this after the mistreatment he had suffered growing up. His blond hair, blue eyes, and handsome looks were a gift of his German lineage. There was an underlying loneliness, a vulnerability to him. There was something childlike and innocent about Elder Schuff.

He looked at me anxiously and said, "I wonder if I can make it through my mission. I'm feeling so bad that I want to go home, but I don't want to seem a failure in the eyes of my family." I answered, "Yes, you can feel much better than this. I will help you so that you can finish your mission comfortably and hopefully with joy."

I placed him on an antidepressant and gradually titrated it upwards. He began to feel calmer and better, but after two months he came to his session in great distress. He burst out, "I am so anxious again." "Why?" I asked. "Did something bad happen?" "No," he responded, "but I can't sleep, I'm really irritable for no reason, and my thoughts are speeded up. I just feel agitated." He looked at me, pleading for an answer.

"Oh, no," I thought, "Elder Schuff is bipolar." I went through all the symptoms on the hypomanic checklist and he answered yes to almost all of them. He said that upon hearing the list, it seemed to him that a maternal uncle and a sister were bipolar as well, suggesting a genetic pattern for the family.

The fifth edition of the American Psychiatric Association's *Diagnostic and Statistical Manual*[iii] lists the diagnostic criteria for a hypomanic episode as follows:

- A distinct period of abnormally and persistently elevated, expansive, or irritable mood and abnormally and persistently increased activity or energy lasting at least four consecutive days and present most of the day, nearly every day.

- During the period of mood disturbance and increased energy and activity, three (or more) of the following symptoms have persisted (four if the mood is only irritable), represent a noticeable change from usual behavior, and have been present to a significant degree:

  - Inflated self-esteem or grandiosity
  - Decreased need for sleep (e.g. feels rested after only three hours of sleep)
  - More talkative than usual or pressure to keep talking
  - Flight of ideas or subjective experience that thoughts are racing

- Distractibility (i.e. attention too easily drawn to unimportant or irrelevant external stimuli), as reported or observed
- Increase in goal-directed activity or psychomotor agitation
- Excessive involvement in activities that have a high potential for painful consequences (e.g. engaging in unrestrained buying sprees, sexual indiscretions, or foolish business investment).

The symptoms of depression are listed in the earlier discussion of Elder Schuff's symptoms and are also addressed in the following chapter on depression.

There are two forms of bipolar disorder: Type I (mania and depression) and Type II (hypomania and depression). Type I affects two percent of the population and type II may affect as much as eight percent of the population according to some studies. The difference is that when people have Bipolar type I disorder, they have psychotic thoughts. For example, one patient reported that she was Jesus Christ nailed to the cross. When I spoke with her the next day, she said she was not Jesus Christ but was His bride and was pregnant with His child. Bipolar type II people by definition do not have psychotic thinking, but they have a higher number of depressive episodes than Bipolar type I, and these episodes can be very debilitating. One study indicated that for Bipolar type II people, the mood disorder usually begins with a depression, and 85 % of the time when their mood is off track, they are depressed.

When a depressed patient is treated with antidepressant medication and hypomanic symptoms appear, the antidepressant is stopped. It takes as long as a month for all the medication to leave the body. If the symptoms of hypomania disappear, they were induced by the medication. If they persist beyond that point, the diagnosis is bipolar illness, and this was the case for Elder Schuff.

When it became apparent that he was bipolar, I had him taper and stop the antidepressant and switched him to bipolar medication. These include mood stabilizers (lithium carbonate, valproic acid, oxycarbamazepine, and lamotrigene) and major tranquilizers (aripiprazole and quetiapine, for example). For Elder Schuff, these medications required many adjustments over the next six months, but eventually on three different medications his mood stabilized and his functioning was much improved.

If someone has never dealt with depression or hypomania, it is hard to understand how difficult it is to endure life. People would advise, "Stop thinking so much about yourself. Go out and serve someone so you will feel better." Or they would offer sympathy, "I know just how you feel. I gave a lesson in Church last Sunday, and it was a real flop." Mood disorders are medical illnesses. When missionaries are depressed all they want to do is stay home and lie in bed, but they have to go out into the world and make contact with others, trying to hide how they really feel. They are representing the Lord's true church and are teaching about the Holy Ghost, but they can't feel it when they are depressed. They are exhausted, unmotivated, negative. Hypomania is also difficult to endure--not the euphoric and grandiose symptoms, but the irritability, intense anxiety, racing thoughts, insomnia, and impulsivity.

I shared the good news with these patients that mood disorders are treatable and that they could return to their best selves and enjoy their missions. Almost all the missionaries I treated for mood disorders chose to stay and were able to regain a level, happy state. When they were feeling well again, I would continue to see them once a month for a fifty minute session until they finished their missions. When people have recently emerged from a serious depression, they are vulnerable to the impact of heightened stress. A difficult companion, a negative ward mission leader, valued investigators who fell away, or trouble in their families at home could trigger a relapse, so I saw them monthly or more often if needed. In those sessions I could give them empathy, understanding, a different perspective, sometimes concrete support like a call to the mission president to request an emergency transfer. We discussed issues from their life before the mission that predisposed or contributed to their depression. I taught them about their illness and how to manage it through the life span. I also adjusted their medications as needed.

There are conditions like Attention Deficit Hyperactivity Disorder that are easy to treat with medicine because once the diagnosis is made and the proper medication and dosage are determined, the patient can often function well for the rest of his life. Bipolar disorder is much more difficult to treat. It usually requires three or four medications to return a patient to a normal mood, and after that it often requires constant attention to keep them stable.

In addition to the use of medication, there are nutraceuticals (foods that provide health benefits) that are also helpful:

- Omega three fatty acids
- Deplin (donates a methyl group in the synthesis of major neurotransmitters, especially important for those with a genetic defect in this rate limiting step of synthesis)
- Vitamin D3 5000 International Units (with a blood level between 30 and 100)
- Vitamin C (Ester C 500 to 1000 mg at bedtime) to lower cortisol levels and thus help maintain Circadian rhythm (day/night cycle)
- Empower Plus, a combination of various vitamins, minerals, and supplements, which has been shown to be effective

I taught my bipolar patients that there are three major factors that destabilize mood in a bipolar person. The first is lack of sleep, the second is stress, and the third is the time of year. Bipolar patients have a genetic predisposition to sleep disturbance. They have trouble falling asleep and then have trouble waking up the next morning. Some of them slip into a pattern of staying up all night and sleeping all the next day, so they try to find jobs that allow them to work later shifts. For missionaries this is a luxury they can't afford, so it becomes important to help them with their sleep difficulties. The use of a Phillips M2 Golite for twenty minutes in the morning helps to keep their Circadian rhythm stable. In general bipolar people are much more stable if their Circadian rhythm is kept in proper order. Destabilizing that will destabilize their mood.

Many bipolar people are sensitive to the rapid shift in the ratio of light to dark that occurs around the spring and fall equinoxes. These shifts affect the Circadian rhythm centers in their brains. When I came to know the individual patterns of a particular patient, I increased his or her medicines several weeks before the equinox and lowered them afterwards.

I taught them about the long term impact of repeated episodes of depression and hypomania or mania. If the mood was not kept stable, there would be long term damage in bipolar patients to areas of the brain involving memory, executive function, and social skills. Young people were not happy to hear that they had a chronic illness which they needed to manage carefully with the assistance of a good psychiatrist, so it was important that they understood the consequences if they chose not to treat their illness. But the message was also that they could probably live normal lives if they did treat it.

I mentioned that Elder Schuff was functioning much better after his mood stabilized, but he still had a high level of anxiety in public. This I felt was not so much bipolar in origin as due to the trauma of his experiences as a child and adolescent. It was also due to the high comorbidity, or overlap, (seventy-five percent) between bipolar disorder and anxiety disorders. I reminded him of how far he had come since those days. He spoke excellent English, was obviously very bright, looked like any other well-groomed missionary in his handsome suit. He had found the Gospel himself and was on his mission without the support of his family. He had written, "I know that the Church of Jesus Christ of Latter-day Saints is God's kingdom here on the earth with prophets and apostles through whom the Lord guides His church. I know of no greater blessing than to be a part of the Lord's kingdom." He was a strong and good man who could hold his head high in any company.

An important part of our work together was our relationship. Perhaps because he was so alone, I felt very protective toward him. There was respect, affection, and hope between us, a delicate and invisible thread that bound us. When he left he gave me a lovely card that said, "Thank you so much. You have solved the mystery of why I am the way I am. Thanks to your wisdom, my life has changed forever and now I can be more useful to the Church and to my family. Love from your patient, Elder Christian Schuff."

Elder Schuff was able to attend college after his mission thanks to the generous support of a member of the Church. When I thought of the boy who went to an English speaking middle school with no knowledge of English, the boy who struggled alone, I was so proud of him. When I spoke with him to ask his permission to tell his story for this book, he was doing well. His mood was stable, he was working, and he was happy.

## Chapter 2: Depression

*I have of late-- but wherefore I know not-- lost all my mirth, forgone all custom of exercises; and indeed it goes so heavily with my disposition that this goodly frame, the earth, seems to be a sterile promontory; this most excellent canopy, the air, look you, this brave o'erhanging firmament, this majestical roof fretted with golden fire, why, it appears no other thing to me than a foul and pestilent congregation of vapours.*

--*Hamlet* by William Shakespeare[iv]

Sister Cameron Snow sat weeping, exhausted, shoulders hunched to defend herself from the pain she was feeling. She was a petite young woman with long brown hair, large hazel eyes, and a narrow face with a pointed chin. She had been out on her mission for seven months and had been feeling worse and worse as the months passed.

"What has caused this depression?" I asked softly, and she shrugged her shoulders. "I'm not sure. It's not the first time I've been depressed, but it's the worst." I responded, "Please tell me about your history so I can understand what this is about."

Sister Snow said that she was the third child of five in a family that struggled financially. Her father was a construction worker who was seasonally employed. The winter months were lean, and then their dinner often consisted of a can of beans. She and her older siblings were sent to visit families that owed her father money for his work, to beg, because they were children, and her father hoped it would soften the hearts of his clients. For her it was humiliating. Her mother was an unhappy and critical woman. Her mother was a twin, and when she was born the umbilical cord was wrapped around her sister's neck, causing anoxia and later profound learning disabilities. Her grandmother blamed her mother for her twin's problems, and the mother grew up as a bitter and angry person. Sister Snow recalled an incident from her own childhood in which an older sister had forcibly taken her toy from her and was playing with it. Cameron ran to tell her mother who responded in a nasty tone, "You are such a tattle-tale. Who cares if she is playing with it?" Her mother pushed her down to the ground. She grew up feeling unimportant, unloved, unhappy.

Her first depression occurred during her adolescence. She lacked confidence and was shy, so making friends was hard for her. She was pretty, so she developed a friendship with a boy named Mark and then started dating him when they were juniors. This was a happy time for her, but as the junior prom approached, Mark did not ask her to go. She found out that he had asked another girl. She thought it might be because he knew she could not afford a prom dress, but she had no one to ask why, and she never found out. They just stopped dating. That is when her first depression began.

The depression lasted through the rest of high school, fueled by her fruitless proximity to Mark and her loneliness. After graduation her depression resolved as she began a new life. She had a series of jobs as a waitress, a salesclerk, and a nanny, saving her money for a mission. Her family members were Mormon but were faint-hearted in their involvement. She would be the first member of her family to go on a mission, and she felt that doing so would give her worth and happiness.

After her twenty first birthday, Cameron submitted her mission papers and received her call to a Spanish speaking part of a United States mission. The MTC was a challenge as she struggled to learn a new language. When she came to the mission, her trainer was difficult. She was a native Spanish speaker who was impatient and controlling. She reminded Sister Snow of her mother, and she began to get depressed again.

"How was she like your mother?" I asked. "She was very critical of the way I spoke Spanish and of my slowness in learning it. I began to be very anxious that during discussions with investigators, she would turn the teaching over to me, and I would only be able to say the most mechanical things. I have a testimony, but I could not even begin to share it." Sister Snow began to sob as she remembered the start to her mission.

"Yes," I nodded, "that sounds like a rough beginning. Were some of your later companions better?" "My next companion was more pleasant, and I began to feel better, but then I was transferred again. I stayed with this companion for two transfers. She was sarcastic and belittling in her humor and often made fun of me, sometimes even mimicking me. I began to feel worse."

Sister Snow said that she could not fall asleep until midnight or 1:00 and woke early. She became more and more exhausted. She lost her appetite and dropped fifteen pounds in three months. She could not concentrate or remember things very well. She began to feel sad, anxious, self-critical, hopeless, and irritable. The mean thoughts she had about herself felt absolutely true. She didn't want to leave the apartment and had no wish to be around other people. Nothing brought her any pleasure or joy, and she could not feel the Holy Ghost. She did not want to kill herself, but said she wouldn't mind if she got hit by a bus and died. She didn't know how she could go on with the rest of her mission.

I said, "You are experiencing a major depression and that is very painful. But I can help you to feel much better, and I think I can help you to enjoy your mission. Would you like to try? Are you willing to stay? It will take a few weeks before you start to feel better, but it will be worth it." She agreed, and we started to work.

Depression is the most common cause of morbidity (including physical illnesses) worldwide. Twenty-five percent of humanity will suffer a depression during their lives. The *Diagnostic and Statistical Manual V*[v] defines depression as follows:

- Five (or more) of the following symptoms have been present during the same two week period and represent a change from previous functioning; at least one of the symptoms is either (1) depressed mood or (2) loss of interest or pleasure.

    - Depressed mood most of the day, nearly every day, as indicated by either subjective report (e.g. feels sad, empty, hopeless) or observation made by others (e.g. appears tearful) (Note: In children and adolescents, can be irritable mood.)
    - Markedly diminished interest or pleasure in all, or almost all, activities most of the day, nearly every day (as indicated by either subjective account or observation)
    - Significant weight loss when not dieting or weight gain (e.g. a change of more than 5% of body weight in a month), or decrease or increase in appetite nearly every day
    - Insomnia or hypersomnia nearly every day
    - Psychomotor agitation or retardation nearly every day (observable by others, not merely subjective feelings of restlessness or being slowed down)
    - Fatigue or loss of energy nearly every day
    - Feelings of worthlessness or excessive or inappropriate guilt (which may be delusional) nearly every day (not merely self-reproach or guilt about being sick)
    - Diminished ability to think or concentrate, or indecisiveness, nearly every day

    - Recurrent thoughts of death (not just fear of dying), recurrent suicidal ideation without a specific plan, or a suicide attempt or a specific plan for committing suicide

- The symptoms cause clinically significant distress or impairment in social, occupational, or other important areas of functioning.

- The episode is not attributable to the physiological effects of a substance or to another medical condition.

- The occurrence of the major depressive episode is not better explained by an illness on the schizophrenia spectrum or other psychotic disorders.

- There has never been a manic episode or a hypomanic episode.

It is important to ask for any history of bipolar disorder in the extended family. If there is such a history, the patient may also be bipolar. If they have never had any symptoms of mania, or its less severe form, which is labeled hypomania, I treat them with antidepressants cautiously, watching for any switch to hypomania. If there has been evidence of bipolar disorder, I use mood stabilizers or major tranquilizers so that the antidepressants don't destabilize their mood further.

There are many causes of depression. Some people have a genetic predisposition to becoming depressed. Others are predisposed to depression by events occurring in the life of their mother while still in her womb. For example, poor nutrition, exposure to toxins, or excessive maternal stress all affect the fetus. Epigenetics also plays a part, that is, negative events may occur over a lifetime that trigger the genes that lead to depression. If people are under stress for a prolonged period, as mentioned before, the increased cortisol can turn off BDNF—brain derived neurotropic factor—which usually protects neurons from injury or degradation when it is active. Some illnesses like mononucleosis include depression as part of that illness. Some medications (e.g. Acutane for acne) can have depression as a side effect. Toxic exposure to substances like tobacco can trigger depression. There is new research that links depression with inflammation. Chronic inflammatory illnesses like rheumatoid arthritis, ulcerative colitis, diabetes, or collagen vascular diseases can lead to depression. New research shows that the inflammatory process releases cytokines—intercellular chemical messengers—that cross into the brain and turn off BDNF. This same process occurs with female abdominal obesity with a BMI over 30. The fat cells release inflammatory cytokines. Heart attacks and strokes are also inflammatory in nature and can be accompanied by depression.

Depression is the brain's way of experiencing pain. One can cut brain tissue with a knife, and it doesn't hurt, but depression is accompanied by elevations of substance P and glutamate in cerebrospinal fluid. These are markers for pain, and when they are elevated, it puts a person at risk for suicide. I was always relieved when a missionary suffering this pain agreed to stay and treat it because I knew they could feel normal again. They could come to love their missions.

Sister Snow was treated with an antidepressant called an SSRI and, after several increases in dose, began to feel better. She still had trouble sleeping, so I added trazadone, the medicine that Missionary Medical insurance allowed me to use to help with insomnia. She could sleep normally, had a return of her appetite, noted improved cognitive function, and no longer felt sad, anxious, hopeless, or irritable. She recovered her energy and felt optimistic about her missionary work again.

Patients do not always respond so readily to medication. Often I have to adjust dosage, augment with a second medication, switch to a different antidepressant, add a mood stabilizer called lamotrigene (which helps with the down side of both unipolar and bipolar mood disorders), or augment with Deplin or thyroid medication. I always recommend adding omega three fatty acids in the form of Megared (krill oil) because this is so helpful in improving mood. I also recommend Vitamin D3 5000 international units monitored with blood tests to keep it in therapeutic range of 30 to 100. I recommend thirty minutes of physical exercise a day. Brisk walking has been shown to significantly help mood.

I informed Sister Snow that once she had responded to medication, she should continue it for a year before tapering and stopping it. Depression is related to BDNF, brain derived neurotropic factor, a central nervous system substance that supports the health of neurons. When it is turned off, by prolonged stress for example, depression results. One of the ways antidepressants work is to turn it back on, but this takes ten to twelve months to accomplish.

I also explained that depression tends to be a recurrent condition. One depression meant that she had a 33% chance of a recurrence. Two depressions meant a 66% chance of recurrence, and three depressions meant a 95% chance. After three depressions people should stay on medication for life. Each recurrence is painful and takes a while to reverse, so it is better to prevent them at that point.

Those who suffer from depression also need to know that untreated depression can damage the brain. It leads to pruning of dendrites, the interconnecting projections of neurons, and to cell death in the hippocampus, the factual memory center of the brain. After five years this atrophy is visible to the naked eye on MRI. Fortunately, these changes are reversible if chronic depression is treated with antidepressants.

For Sister Snow, it helped that her latest transfer had paired her with a gentle, accepting companion, but knowing that this could change again, I wanted to strengthen her to withstand blows from others. I asked her to note down every critical thought she had about herself and report them to me. She said, "That's hard. There are so many of them every day. I think I am a bad missionary, that I don't have enough courage, that my testimony is not strong enough, that I can't think fast enough, that other sisters have a more creative way of teaching, that I don't have as much love for people as other sisters do..."

"Hold on," I said. "That sounds so discouraging. You also ran through that list so fast that it sounds like you have practiced that speech many times in your head. You are much less depressed now and have the option of thinking positively, but this seems to be the default setting of your brain."

Sister Snow admitted that this was a habit of many years duration. "Is there a voice connected with this list?" I asked. "Oh, yes, it definitely is my mother's voice. I can see her face. Angry, yelling, scary." "Were you ever angry back?" "No, she would have hit me. I did run away when I was twelve. I ran to my neighbor's house and spent the night in her garage. She never knew. But I went back the next day. Hungry, I guess." She looked ashamed at her failed attempt to escape. I said, "What has become of that anger?" "I guess I have buried it. I have built a shell around myself so no one will know how angry I am inside. I try to be nice so people will like me."

"But they aren't always nice back, like some of your companions. Let's think about ways you might have stood up to them. How about your first companion?" Sister Snow said, "Well, she always left the dishes for me. I wanted to tell her she should do them half the time, but I was afraid." I responded, "So you were just silently angry. I think that is a recipe for depression. You don't have to be like your mother when you express anger or set limits on someone else's misbehavior. Maybe you are afraid you will turn into her if you get angry. You can be matter of fact but determined. While we have time together, it would be good if you could experiment and tell me how it goes. It will take courage, but it is worth it."

As Sister Snow and I worked on her difficulty with anger--her own and others'--she began to dismantle her shell and to feel more connected to her companions and her investigators. She gained confidence, taught with more power, and began to see herself as a creative person with good ideas. She began to have hope for her future, that when she became a wife and mother she wouldn't have to be just like her mother and grandmother.

When people came to me in the midst of a depression, there was a sameness about them. I always wondered, "What is the real personality of this patient?" As they felt better, I got to see their sense of humor, their spiritual depth, their enthusiasm for life. But even though depression robbed them of their personality and made them flat, each person brought a unique set of problems and gifts for us to unravel. It was so rewarding to help missionaries remain on their missions, to see them overcome their pain and blossom spiritually. They grew to love their missions.

Sister Snow finished her mission and went home. Her missionary letters had a powerful influence on her older sister, who had come back to full activity in the Church. They moved in together and, with the emotional support of her sister, Sister Snow was able to complete a program that allowed her to become a marriage and family counselor. Her experience with depression gave her a deep understanding of the pain and stress people suffered. She became an excellent counselor and eventually a wonderful wife and mother.

## Chapter 3: Anxiety Disorders

*There were also dreadful, pouncing seizures of anxiety. One bright day on a walk through the woods with my dog I heard a flock of Canada geese honking high above trees ablaze with foliage; ordinarily a sight and sound that would have exhilarated me, the flight of birds caused me to stop, riveted with fear, and I stood stranded there, helpless, shivering.*

--*Darkness Visible* by William Styron[vi]

Elder Trent Fulton loved alternative rock music, fireworks, and described himself as the problem kid in the family. He had been an angry, depressed adolescent, but this was not obvious from his appearance. Like most missionaries, he looked angelic in his suit, white shirt, and name tag. He had short brown hair with green eyes, beautiful large eyes, but strangely lacking eyelashes. He was of medium height and slender build and sat quietly on my sofa. He had been on his mission for sixteen months, so he had eight months to go.

"How can I help you?" I asked as we settled down to work. "I have been getting more and more anxious," he answered. "I'm afraid my body is taking the brunt of it. I pull out my eyelashes and eyebrows, grind my teeth at night, my back is killing me, and I have acid reflux. I can't wake up in the morning, so I'm tired a lot." Medically he had trichotillomania (hair pulling), bruxism (teeth grinding), muscle spasms, and gastroesophageal reflux. Underlying these manifestations, he had generalized anxiety disorder, or GAD.

He had begun treatment for anxiety when he was twelve years old. He had been on a variety of antidepressants (Luvox, Paxil, Prozac, and Effexor) and benzodiazepines (Valium, Xanax, Ativan, and Klonopin) before his mission. Missionary Medical doesn't allow the use of benzodiazepines on missions because of their potential for habituation and abuse, so he was only on Effexor, a dual action antidepressant that affects serotonin and norepinephrine, which he had started five years before his mission. His father and two of his paternal aunts also used benzodiazepines for chronic anxiety.

Elder Fulton was the oldest of six children. His siblings were talented musically, gifted academically, and good natured. His father was kind, musical, athletic, and smart. He composed music, sang, and played piano and guitar. He ran his own business, was active in the Church, was a good husband, and a loving, sensitive father. He never lost his temper. His parents had a very good marriage, and he never saw them fight. His mother was empathic, creative, patient, and a good homemaker. She was a teacher before he was born but stayed at home to raise her family.

Trent Fulton had Attention Deficit Hyperactivity Disorder in addition to his anxiety. He began taking Adderall, a stimulant medication for ADHD, during his junior year in high school. It caused an increase in his trichotillomania (hair pulling), so he used small doses. He went to a community college for two years and did well in science classes, but he got depressed and had to drop a semester. He transferred to another school for a semester and then came on his mission.

On his mission he had a resurgence of his anxiety. He said the anxiety was due to the buildup of ordinary mission stresses rather than any one precipitant. The source of Elder Fulton's anxiety was more internal than external. He had GAD, one form of the anxiety disorders, which is defined by the DSM V[vii] as follows:

- Excessive anxiety and worry, occurring more days than not for at least six months, about a number of events or activities (such as work or school performance)
- The individual finds it difficult to control the worry

- The anxiety and worry are associated with three (or more) of the following six symptoms:
    1. Restlessness or feeling keyed up or on edge.
    2. Being easily fatigued.
    3. Difficulty concentrating or mind going blank.
    4. Irritability
    5. Muscle tension
    6. Sleep disturbance (difficulty falling or staying asleep, or restless, unsatisfying sleep)

- The anxiety, worry, or physical symptoms cause clinically significant distress or impairment in social, occupational, or other important areas of functioning

The essential feature of generalized anxiety disorder is excessive anxiety and worry about a number of events or activities. The intensity, duration, or frequency of the anxiety and worry is out of proportion to the actual likelihood or impact of the anticipated event. The individual finds it difficult to control the worry and to keep worrisome thoughts from interfering with attention to tasks at hand. Adults with generalized anxiety disorder often worry about every day, routine life circumstances, such as possible job responsibilities, health and finances, the health of family members, misfortune to their children, or minor matters. During the course of the disorder, the focus of worry may shift from one concern to another.

Several features distinguish generalized anxiety disorder from nonpathological anxiety. First, the worries associated with generalized anxiety disorder are excessive and typically interfere significantly with psychosocial functioning, whereas the worries of everyday life are not excessive and are perceived as more manageable and may be put off when more pressing matters arise.

GAD affects nine percent of the population across the life span. Females are twice as likely as males to experience GAD. The symptoms tend to be chronic and to wax and wane throughout life, but it is rare to be fully free of it. GAD doesn't usually appear before adolescence. When it begins, the worries are about school and sports performance; for older adults the worries center around the well being of family or their own physical health.

Behavioral inhibition and harm avoidance have been associated with GAD. No environmental factors have been identified as specific to GAD. (Remember the positive family history that Elder Fulton gave.) One-third of the risk of experiencing GAD is genetic, and these genetic factors also predispose to other forms of anxiety and to major depression.

Excessive worrying impairs the individual's capacity to do things quickly and efficiently, whether at home or at work. The worrying takes time and energy; the associated symptoms of muscle tension and feeling keyed up or on edge, tiredness, difficulty concentrating, and disturbed sleep contribute to the impairment.

Intense anxiety is a very painful emotion. Some people who have both anxiety and depression tell me depression is easier to bear.

Other anxiety disorders listed in the DSM V include:

- Separation anxiety
- Selective mutism (usually a childhood disorder)
- Phobias (specific, social, or agoraphobia)
- Panic disorder

Although they were not a part of Elder Fulton's difficulties, many missionaries have been troubled with panic attacks. These are very disturbing events. The DSM V[viii] diagnosis is given below:

> A panic attack is an abrupt surge of intense fear or intense discomfort that reaches a peak within minutes, and during which time four (or more) of the following symptoms occur:

- Palpitations, pounding heart, or accelerated heart rate
- Sweating
- Trembling or shaking
- Sensations of shortness of breath or smothering
- Chest pain or discomfort
- Nausea or abdominal distress
- Feeling dizzy, unsteady, lightheaded or faint
- Chills or heat sensations
- Paresthesias (numbness or tingling sensations)
- Derealization (feelings of unreality) or depersonalization (being detached from oneself)
- Fear of losing control or going crazy
- Fear of dying

Panic attacks can be present in many disorders: bipolar disorder, posttraumatic stress disorder, depression, other anxiety disorders, impulse control disorders, or substance abuse. Sometimes panic attacks are triggered by hyperventilation, that is, rapid and shallow breathing from the apex of the lungs. This changes the oxygen/carbon dioxide ratio and is read by a part of the brain called the locus ceruleous, the fear center of the brain. When this fires, the symptoms of a panic attack ensue. The symptoms last from fifteen to forty-five minutes and are genuinely terrifying events. Once people have experienced one, they develop anticipatory anxiety that they will have another.

A patient came in to report that she had a lovely lunch with her friends, and at the end of it she had a most unexpected panic attack. I asked her if she was wearing a tight belt, and her eyes widened as she answered that she was indeed. As her stomach swelled with her lunch, the belt constricted her deep breathing.

Another patient went hiking on the Appalachian Trail with a friend. He did well for the first two weeks, but after a short rest at his aunt's house, he developed panic attacks on the trail and had to come home. I asked him if he had changed equipment at his aunt's home, and he said that he had exchanged his back pack for a new one. Upon questioning, he recalled that the new back pack had tight shoulder straps that constricted his breathing. He had no panic attacks when he wasn't wearing it.

A third patient had panic attacks after he fell on the ice and broke two ribs. The pain had constricted his breathing.

Another patient had his first panic attack at his grandfather's funeral. He had a strong testimony of the Gospel and a belief in the Resurrection, but confronted with death for the first time, he felt like he was falling down an endless black tunnel, falling through the universe. He began to hyperventilate, and this triggered a panic attack. Unlike the previous examples, this needed work in psychotherapy to explore his fears and find comfort for them.

It is a different matter if people wake from a sound sleep in the midst of a panic attack. This is the result of neither hyperventilation nor psychodynnamics but rather from an overreactive locus ceruleous.

When I treat people with panic attacks, I tell them that they need to breathe deeply and slowly (from fifteen breaths per minute, our usual rate, down to four per minute.) They need to breathe from the bottom of their lungs, expanding the bottom of their rib cage. By disciplining their breathing, they reset the oxygen/carbon dioxide ratio and calm the locus ceruleous. If they can do this early in the cycle of a panic attack, they can reverse it.

Patients can also treat recurrent panic disorder with antidepressants, which treat anxiety as well as depression. The medication is taken daily to prevent attacks, not in the midst of an attack. It is not helpful to use benzodiazepines like Xanax because they take fifteen minutes to take effect, and by that time most panic attacks are resolving.

Sometimes panic attacks lead to the development of agoraphobia. I treated a woman late in the course of her illness who had a history of panic attacks. They had occurred at the post office, in the grocery store, and at the mall. After each attack, she avoided that place in the future and her world narrowed. Eventually she became housebound and went on disability. This points to the importance of early diagnosis and treatment of panic disorder.

There are many types of phobias, but the most common is social phobia which affects about fifteen percent of the population in the United States across the life span. This diagnosis involves an intense fear of being judged, especially in social situations. I had a patient whose mother abandoned her at the age of two. She went to live with her father and step-mother who eventually had four children of their own. My patient was treated like a servant of the family by her emotionally cold and abusive step-mother. As an adult, this patient was extremely anxious in social situations. She gave a dinner party and was terrified far in advance that her guests would be critical of her home, table settings, food, appearance, or conversation at dinner. Criticism was at the top of her list of fears. We approached this both with insight oriented psychotherapy and with cognitive behavioral therapy.

Considering the intense discomfort of anxiety disorders, I was eager to help missionaries feel calmer. Elder Fulton came to therapy distressed by his companion. He said, “He talks behind my back, sulks if he doesn’t get his way, and orders me around.” The stress was amplifying his GAD and his hair pulling. I asked him how he was responding, and he answered, “I am not responding. I am just withdrawing and shutting down. Nobody ever did that in my family.” I suggested that he needed to confront this companion, to tell him he had heard from other elders at the last zone conference that he was talking behind his back. I asked what his companion had been saying, and from his response I could tell that his companion was envious of his excellent teaching skills and strong testimony. I said, "It sounds like you also need to build him up, to tell him good things about himself to bolster his self-esteem. Can you think of any good qualities?" That was his only really difficult companion. Elder Fulton told me that both mission presidents he served under were careful to give him good companions who were easy to get along with because they wanted to lessen his stress.

Elder Fulton said he felt anxious about fulfilling goals of the mission. For example, he and his companion were supposed to spend a certain number of hours per week tracting. He found this easiest when he was a senior companion and had some control of the schedule. He could mix harder tasks with easier ones. Elder Fulton had his own ways of lessening stress. At times he needed to take a step back to regain his composure and confidence. He would lie down to meditate or take a short nap at lunch, especially if he was tired or stressed. Because of his strong musical background, it helped to listen to classical guitar. Positive correspondence with family and friends was also helpful.

We treated his GAD with Effexor 150 mg ER, and this was increased to 225 mg after a month to help lessen the anxiety. He stayed on this comfortably for the rest of his mission.

A short time after I began to treat Elder Fulton, his mission president called to tell me that Elder Fulton was not using his Friday morning planning time to organize for the coming week. Instead he was playing around. The mission president had been pressuring him to settle down but to no avail. This was a symptom of his Attention Deficit Hyperactivity Disorder. I began treatment with Concerta, a milder stimulant since he had an increase in his hair pulling when he used Adderall in high school. Concerta didn't work, so I tried Strattera, a nonstimulant second tier medicine, but it had unacceptable side effects. Adderall XR made him feel flat, so we switched to short acting Adderall 10 mg twice a day. This was successful in treating the ADHD and did not worsen the hair pulling, so he remained on this through the rest of his mission.

As previously mentioned, his second comorbidity was trichotillomania, or hair pulling. This is a disorder that ranges from mild to severe. I had one patient who was completely bald and wore a hat to disguise it. It is listed in the DSM V as an OCD related disorder, and like OCD it is much worse under stress. Elder Fulton noticed that increased stress led to increased pulling of his eyelashes and eyebrows. There is no single group of medicines that helps trichotillomania. Patients respond to a variety of medicines, but it is unpredictable and personal. I treated my bald patient with fifteen different medicines from every major group and none helped much. She did best over summer breaks. Fortunately Elder Fulton had a mild case, and this was not a focus of our treatment.

As Elder Fulton thought about his spiritual progress on his mission he described it as a gradual process. As he read the scriptures and prayed daily, he felt more in tune with his Heavenly Father. He bore his testimony frequently and found it growing stronger with repetition. He found peace, comfort, and direction.

After Elder Fulton completed his mission he went on to graduate from college. He married a lovely woman five years ago, and they are expecting their first child this spring. He has applied to programs to become a pharmacist, his dream for many years. He is doing very well.

## Chapter 4: Obsessive Compulsive Disorder (OCD)

*I am plagued by doubts. What if everything is an illusion and nothing exists? In that case, I definitely overpaid for my carpets.*

--*Without Feathers* by Woody Allen[ix]

When I met Elder Jack Singer, he had been on his mission for seven months. His mission had started off well enough with an excellent trainer whom he respected, but his next companion had been tough, critical, hard to please. His confidence had begun to falter, his old insomnia returned, and he could feel himself becoming more anxious. With his third companion, he had a serious bike accident from which he was still recovering. It had made him still more anxious, and that led to some strange thoughts.

"Elder Singer," I questioned, "what do you mean by strange thoughts?" Elder Singer looked down at his folded hands, his green eyes avoiding mine. He began quietly, "Well, when we went to the temple last week, I looked at a picture of the Savior and saw a cigarette hanging out of his mouth. I couldn't get it out of my head the whole time we were in the temple. Then over the weekend I started thinking I sold my soul to the devil." I acknowledged how disturbing these thoughts could be, then asked if he had had these or similar thoughts before. They had started at eight years of age when he was standing at the beach. Suddenly he had the awful thought that he had sold his soul to the devil. As a child he would tap three fingers on his other arm to chase the thought away, but it always came back. Finally it faded after several years.

I asked him if he had told anyone about these thoughts. He had shared them with his parents and was taken to a child psychiatrist who made the diagnosis of Obsessive Compulsive

Disorder and treated him with therapy and an antidepressant, citalopram. He recovered and was fine for a long time. His parents were supportive; indeed his mother had OCD and had to come home early from her mission for obsessions and extreme perfectionism.

His family gave him a good start in life. His parents had a good marriage with little conflict. Neither one was much of a disciplinarian, but the children were well behaved. He was the oldest of four sons, and they got along well. His father was a hard worker, active in the Church, but was not good at handling money. They were often in debt, and this gave Jack cause to worry. He identified closely with his father, who was a singer. Jack was involved in theater and singing in high school, and his parents attended his performances regularly.

His mother was patient, loving, and supportive. She worked full time, cooked occasionally, and loved to watch movies. Her extended family struggled with depression and OCD, consistent with the fact that OCD is a genetic disorder. As Elder Singer described his family to me, I heard some cause for anxiety but also much that would contribute to a sense of security and to the development of good social skills.

Jack Singer did well until his senior year of high school. That year he was taking hard classes, working part time, and was in the school play. The stress set off another round of OCD and, this time, a serious depression. He resumed treatment. He went off to college in the fall, but his illnesses got in his way, and he did not do well that semester. He decided to work until he went on his mission.

Obsessive Compulsive Disorder is defined in the *Diagnostic and Statistical Manual of Mental Disorders, Fifth Edition*[x] as the presence of obsessions, compulsions, or both.

- Obsessions are defined by:
  - Recurrent and persistent thoughts, urges, or images that are experienced, at some time

during the disturbance, as intrusive and unwanted, and that in most individuals cause marked anxiety or distress.
    - The individual attempts to ignore or suppress such thoughts, urges, or images, or to neutralize them with some other thought or action (i.e. by performing a compulsion).

- Compulsions are defined by:
    - Repetitive behaviors (e.g. hand washing, ordering, checking) or mental acts (e.g. praying, counting, repeating words silently) that the individual feels driven to perform in response to an obsession or according to rules that must be applied rigidly.
    - The behaviors or mental acts are aimed at preventing or reducing anxiety or distress or preventing some dreaded event or situation; however, these behaviors or mental acts are not connected in a realistic way with what they are designed to neutralize or prevent, or are clearly excessive.

- The obsessions or compulsions are time consuming (e.g. take more than one hour per day) or cause clinically significant distress or impairment in social, occupational, or other important areas of functioning.

OCD has a genetic component and is frequently comorbid with Attention Deficit Hyperactivity Disorder, depression, and tic disorder. It is not rare; the prevalence is 1.2% of the population.

I have seen many people with OCD over the years. Their obsessions can include:

- Contamination obsessions and cleaning compulsions (for example, a teenage girl who felt that chlorine from the swimming pool was damaging to her, so she would wash her bathing suit, towel, carrying bag, and if the bag touched her bed, all her linens as well)
- Symmetry obsessions and repeating, ordering, and counting compulsions (for example, the child who had to count the tiles in the shower in patterns of numbers, and if he got off track he had to start all over, making him late for school because his showers took so long)
- Forbidden or taboo thoughts that are aggressive or sexual, or religious obsessions and compulsions (for example, a man who was afraid he would stab his wife whom he loved dearly)
- Fears of harm to oneself or others (for example, the young woman who was afraid she was dragging a body under her car, so she had to pull over and check under the car frequently)

OCD can change forms over time. Symptoms can fall under several or many of the headings. Those who suffer can be free of symptoms for many years and then have a recurrence, especially during times of stress.

It is hard enough for anyone to have OCD, which can interfere with school or work and cause terrible anxiety, but it is even harder for missionaries. For those OCD missionaries who strive to be perfect, OCD brings misery because they are so critical of the smallest failure. One of my OCD missionaries was instructed upon leaving the

MTC to never waste a moment of his mission. He did not need this advice. He lived his whole life that way, so he pushed himself until he was working in a haze of exhaustion and anxiety. I told him that advice was for the slackers, not for OCD perfectionists.

Elder Singer also struggled to tell the difference between his OCD thoughts and the inspiration of the Holy Ghost. He could not differentiate them and was not sure he could follow the ideas that came into his head. I remembered a missionary I had worked with earlier in my career. He also had OCD and felt that the Holy Ghost was telling him to go home early from his mission. I told him that the Holy Ghost inspires us to make spiritual progress. His messages are for good. That seems to me to be a valid measure: if thoughts refine our spirit and suggest a good course, they are from the Spirit, not illness.

When a missionary with OCD has made a moral mistake before his mission, it becomes difficult for him to forgive himself. I worked with Elder White, a young man who had confessed his transgressions to the bishop and stake president and repented of them. He confessed them again in the MTC, and then in the mission field he confessed them to his mission president. He had been referred to me for symptoms of OCD, and he told me of the thought that would give him no peace: "I haven't confessed well enough. I left out some of the details. Maybe I won't be forgiven, so I had better confess again." As he revealed this fear, he clenched his fists on his knees and looked at me with anguish. Each time he would confess, he would feel relief for a little while, but then the pressure to confess again would start to build. This is typical of OCD, and the repetition strengthens the disorder. I told Elder White that he had to resist the urge to confess yet again and called his mission president to share my knowledge of this OCD pattern. I asked him not to allow Elder White to confess anymore. He agreed to this and left it to us to work it out in therapy.

I taught Elder White a behavioral approach to help with OCD. It is simple to say but hard to do. The first step is to acknowledge, "The thought or behavior is not me; it is my OCD." The second step is, "And the more I think or do it, the stronger it gets." Step three is to put the mind elsewhere, somewhere detailed but neutral. People can think of what they want to fix for dinner and whether they have all the ingredients they will need, a favorite movie scene, a poem they have memorized. It is a personal choice, but it needs to replace the obsession. This is very difficult at first, but as the person practices, it gets easier, lasts longer, and weakens the OCD.

OCD can be so severe that it is helpful to use medications at first. This helps to lessen the intensity of the OCD with its attendant anxiety so that the person can master the behavioral approach. After several months the medication can often be tapered and stopped. The usual choice would be an SSRI antidepressant like Prozac, Zoloft, or Lexapro, but for severe cases the major tranquilizers like Abilify or Seroquel can be helpful. The major tranquilizers are for short term use because if they are used longer they can cause tardive dyskinesia, a permanent movement disorder.

Elder White was treated with Lexapro and was responding well, but he still had great difficulty with tracting. He could not bear the rejection of doors slammed in his face, took it personally, and became unbearably anxious when it was time to tract. I taught him to do deep breathing for five minutes before he and his companion left the apartment. This was somewhat helpful, but he remained anxious about tracting, so I suggested that he set goals (knock on ten doors and then reward himself with a short break). Three more months dragged by, and then he was assigned to an understanding, supportive companion that made tracting much better. Elder White came in the following month and reported that he was more relaxed and doing well. He had changed his approach during tracting: he had decided to relate to those he contacted as people first before introducing the Gospel. This worked wonders for several months until the mission president introduced a new technique. He wanted the missionaries to do "lightning strikes" with street contacts, to approach people and immediately share a gospel message. Elder White was always an obedient missionary, but this was the reverse of the solution he had painstakingly worked out for months. He tried it for several weeks and returned for his next session in great distress. The anxiety of the lightning strikes had triggered his OCD once again. I called the mission president, explained the problem, and was relieved when he gave his consent for Elder White to drop this approach and return to his own successful method. It worked. His OCD quieted down.

I have never seen a missionary develop OCD for the first time on a mission, but it often seems to get worse when they come on a mission. Missions are stressful. My son commented that he gave up everything but his religion when he went on his mission--school, job, clothing style, hair style, girlfriend, movies, music, sports, family. Even his name was different since no one called him by his first name. It is hard to relieve stress minus the outlets one developed before the mission.

Missions are also stressful because of the responsibility for finding those who will accept the Gospel, the relentless and exhausting pace of the work, and the obedience to rules not of one's own making. On top of these stressors, add difficult companions, homesickness, frustration with promising investigators who drop the Church, and often the struggle to learn a new language and teach subtle concepts in that language.

Stress triggers OCD, but as missionaries grapple with its challenge, they develop greater faith because they must turn to the Lord for help. They receive inspired Priesthood blessings. They work in spite of their difficulties. They grow stronger. Together we treated their OCD, so none of them went home early. They were able to gain the wonderful spiritual blessings that come from serving a full mission.

## Chapter 5: Attention Deficit Hyperactivity Disorder (ADHD)

*Attention deficit disorder, or ADD, is a misleading name for an intriguing kind of mind. ADD is a name for a collection of symptoms, some positive, some negative. For many people, ADD is not a disorder but a trait, a way of being in the world. When it impairs their lives, then it becomes a disorder. But once they learn to manage its disorderly aspects, they can take full advantage of the many talents and gifts embedded in this sparkling kind of mind.*

*Delivered from Distraction* by Hallowell and Ratey[xi]

I welcomed my next patient, Elder Thomas Sommers, an enthusiastic, high energy young man. He bounded up my steep staircase two steps at a time and sat perched on the sofa, legs crossed with one foot bouncing rapidly. His internal engine was in high gear. He had hair that stood straight up as if an electric current had exited his body at the top of his head. He had a mischievous grin and a sparkle in his eye that announced him as one of God's jesters. Speaking quickly, he told me that he and his companion and their roommates had been bored the past week and had entertained themselves by throwing some old bikes off the balcony of their third floor apartment into the yard below to see who could throw them the farthest. They would throw them, run down and retrieve them, and start the fun all over again. The game was his idea. I thought, "Aren't we lucky to have such a high spirited, energetic young man in our mission?"

I was treating Elder Sommers for attention deficit hyperactivity disorder (ADHD). He had not been diagnosed with this before his mission and had been frustrated that on his mission he couldn't concentrate when reading the scriptures or doing his studies. He could not keep his mind on discussions, and when his companion handed off the lessons to him, he had no idea what they had been talking about or what he should say. He quickly became bored with their daily routine and felt trapped without his usual outlets of sports and computer games. He could not pay attention in zone conference or church meetings. He didn't like to be told what to do, which included obeying the mission rules. He liked companions who were similar to him, playful and mischievous, but he intensely disliked companions who were driven, rule-oriented, and serious. They made him feel like a slacker because they were all work and no play.

As a child, Elder Sommers had been an average student. He didn't like homework. He told his mother that it was really schoolwork, so he should do it at school and not at home. Home was for playing, running, climbing, jumping, riding his bike, moving as much as possible. He was a creative child and loved to build things out of pieces of wood, string, old nails, and cardboard. One time he disassembled their brick patio to build a fortress, much to his mother's dismay. When he was doing something that interested him, he could pay attention for hours, but if something did not engage him, he would rush through it and often not complete it. He did not manage time well and was usually late for everything except meals.

As he grew older, he did not write down the assignments given by the teachers, did not bring home the books he needed to do his work, could not settle down to do homework, or if he did, could not do it without his mother by his side to help him stay on task. It took him three times longer to do his work than most other boys in class. If he did finish his homework, he often did not put it in his backpack to take to school. If he did get it to school, he would forget to hand it in. His mother would find it months later crumpled up in the bottom of his backpack. Long term projects were the worst. He would forget about them until the last few days and then do them in a rush. Because he was creative, he could have done much better if only he had given himself enough time. Procrastination was his middle name. He was on the receiving end of many lectures and punishments. His parents did not realize that he responded much better to reward than punishment.

Although his grades were mediocre in elementary school and slid downhill as he moved through high school, he had close friends. He was funny. He could quote whole scenes from movies in the voices of the characters. He was irreverent in his humor and liked to provoke others, especially his siblings, but he was also so much fun with his spontaneity and love of adventure that people wanted to be with him. He was fearless because he did not think ahead. He could have a flash temper, but it subsided quickly.

As he became an adolescent, he found that playing computer games helped him feel less bored, more peaceful. It became a further source of conflict with his parents that he spent hours playing on the computer and procrastinated his work until the end of the day. When they suggested that he do his work first and use the game as a reward, he quickly answered, "Oh, I don't do things that way." In spite of his impulsive and provocative nature, he did not get into serious trouble as an adolescent and was able to go on a mission. He had come from a good family and a fine ward in which he had a group of friends who were also avoiding alcohol and drugs as they prepared for missions. In this he was very fortunate.

On his mission he was without his usual outlets and had to confront his limitations. As time passed he began to get depressed. He was referred to me for that, not for ADHD, but as he gave me his history it was clear that his unrecognized, untreated ADHD was the source of his difficulty. I used the following diagnostic criteria from the DSM V:[xii]

- A persistent pattern of inattention and/or hyperactivity-impulsivity that interferes with functioning or development, as characterized by inattention and/or hyperactivity and impulsivity:

- Inattention: Six (or more) of the following symptoms have persisted for at least six months to a degree that is inconsistent with developmental level or that negatively impacts directly on social and academic/occupational activities:
    - Often fails to give close attention to details or makes careless mistakes in schoolwork, at work, or during other activities (e.g., overlooks or misses details, work is inaccurate)
    - Often has difficulty sustaining attention in tasks or play activities (e.g. has difficulty remaining focused during lectures, conversation, or length reading).
    - Often does not seem to listen when spoken to directly (e.g. mind seems elsewhere, even in the absence of any obvious distraction)
    - Often does not follow through on instructions and fails to finish schoolwork, chores, or duties in the workplace (e.g. starts tasks but quickly loses focus and is easily sidetracked)
    - Often has difficulty organizing tasks and activities (e.g. difficulty managing sequential tasks; difficulty keeping materials and belongings in order; messy, disorganized work; has poor time management; fails to meet deadlines)
    - Often avoids, dislikes, or is reluctant to engage in tasks that require sustained mental effort (e.g. schoolwork or homework; for older

adolescents and adults, preparing reports, completing forms, reviewing lengthy papers)
  - Often loses things necessary for tasks or activities (e.g. school materials, pencils, books, tools, wallets, keys, paperwork, eyeglasses, mobile telephones)
  - Is often easily distracted by extraneous stimuli (for older adolescents and adults, may include unrelated thoughts)
  - Is often forgetful in daily activities (e.g. doing chores, running errands; for older adolescents and adults, returning calls, paying bills, keeping appointments)

- Hyperactivity and impulsivity: Six (or more) of the following symptoms have persisted for at least six months to a degree that is inconsistent with developmental level and that negatively impacts directly on social and academic/occupational activities:
  - Often fidgets with or taps hands or feet or squirms in seat
  - Often leaves seat in situations when remaining seated is expected (e.g. leaves his or her place in the classroom, in the office or other workplace, or in other situations that require remaining in place)
  - Often runs about or climbs in situations where it is inappropriate (Note: in adolescents or adult, may be limited to feeling restless.)
  - Often unable to play or engage in leisure activities quietly

- Is often "on the go," acting as if "driven by a motor" (e.g. is unable to be or uncomfortable being still for extended time, as in restaurants, meetings; may be experienced by others as being restless or difficult to keep up with)
- Often talks excessively
- Often blurts out an answer before a question has been completed (e.g. completes people's sentences; cannot wait for turn in conversation)
- Often has difficulty waiting his or her turn (e.g. while waiting in line)
- Often interrupts or intrudes on others (e.g. butts into conversation, games, or activities; may start using other people's things without asking or receiving permission; for adolescents and adults, may intrude into or take over what others are doing)

- Several inattentive or hyperactive-impulsive symptoms were present prior to age twelve years.

- Several inattentive or hyperactive-impulsive symptoms are present in two or more settings (e.g., at home, school, or work; with friends or relatives; in other activities).

- There is clear evidence that the symptoms interfere with, or reduce the quality of, social, academic, or occupational functioning.

- The symptoms do not occur exclusively during the course of schizophrenia or another psychotic disorder and are not better explained by another mental disorder (e.g., mood disorder, anxiety disorder, dissociative disorder, personality disorder, substance intoxication or withdrawal).

Manifestations of the disorder must be present in more than one setting (e.g. home and school, work). Confirmation of substantial symptoms across settings typically cannot be done accurately without consulting informants who have seen the individual in those settings. Typically, symptoms vary depending on context within a given setting. Signs of the disorder may be minimal or absent when the individual is receiving frequent rewards for appropriate behavior, is under close supervision, is in a novel setting, is engaged in especially interesting activities, has consistent external stimulation (e.g. via electronic screens), or is interacting in one-on-one situations.

I used these criteria in diagnosing ADHD and also administered several standard checklists which I further used for reference and comparison as I treated the disorder. Any time I evaluated a missionary, I got his or her permission to talk with the mission president and parents to gather more history, explain the diagnosis, and tell how I planned to treat the difficulty. When I called Elder Sommer's parents to explain his diagnosis, they responded that his father and two of his four siblings sounded like they also had ADHD. That made sense as it is a genetic disorder. They were willing to let me treat him.

ADHD is not rare. Probably 8% of the population has this condition. There must be many missionaries who don't know they have ADHD who serve successful missions. There are inherent patterns in missions that are useful in helping with this condition and are part of the behavioral approach I teach my ADHD patients. For example, there is a built in structure that helps a missionary to organize his day and week. He has a planning session with his companion each week, sometimes each day, which helps him organize his priorities and his time. He has a notebook with the information about investigators, schedules, goals. He has a companion, another person who works with him and to whom he is accountable. Missions teach organizational skills and self-discipline and give a higher purpose to life that motivates people. In addition, I teach missionaries with ADHD to use reminders like post-it notes displayed in prominent places like the refrigerator, to always put their keys in the same place, to put their medicine next to their toothbrush so they remember to take it every day. I encourage my ADHD missionaries to continue to apply these skills after they go home.

According to Dr. Ned Hallowell and Dr. John Ratey, psychiatrists who have written several excellent books about ADHD, physical exercise promotes sustained attention, the ability to stay alert and remain on task. They recommend that if an ADHD person finds himself becoming spacey, he can reset his brain with a short burst of exercise like doing twenty jumping jacks or running up and down stairs a few times. They recommend regular exercise on a daily basis to promote health in our body as well as our brain.

Nutrition is also important. While excessive intake of sugar does not cause ADHD, it can make ADHD people more hyper. A good diet rich in protein, fresh fruits and vegetables provides an even, steady flow of energy that helps the brain function better. In addition, omega three fatty acids are extremely helpful because they are used as building blocks in cell walls and the walls of mitochondria, the power houses of all cells including those in the brain. These walls are composed of lipids, and the nature of our lipid intake has changed dramatically over the last century. As we take in ever more processed foods with omega six fatty acids in them and consume less of the fresh foods that carry omega threes, these walls become less permeable. Our brains work better if we supplement our diets with omega three fatty acids, and this can be done most easily with fish oil capsules or krill oil capsules. MegaRed is a good source because it is made from krill and doesn't have a fishy aftertaste.

Another important supplement is called Deplin, or methylated folate. It donates a methyl group in the metabolism of central nervous system neurotransmitters like serotonin, norepinephrine, and dopamine. This is especially important in those with a genetic make-up which lacks the enzyme that confers this ability, but anyone can benefit from it. Dopamine and norepinephrine are central to executive functioning, and in part ADHD is caused by a failure to release dopamine in the frontal lobe of the brain when confronted with tasks that seem boring. Deplin helps by increasing the supply of these neurotransmitters.

Medication is another extremely important part of ADHD treatment. The behavioral approaches can help to organize life, but the only effective way to treat wandering attention is with medication. The most effective medications are the stimulants like Ritalin, Concerta, Dexedrine, Adderall, and Vyvanse. Each of these has its own personality, but they all work by stimulating the release of dopamine in the frontal lobe of the brain. If the medications are effective, they help with the ability to jump start the brain, inhibit wandering attention and thus make work more efficient, help break big tasks into smaller parts so they seem less overwhelming, prioritize tasks, and complete work. The medication also helps to control temper, lessen provocative behavior, and even out mood.

One mother wrote, "I wanted to let you know my daughter is seeing a wonderful psychiatrist and since she started medication it is just like you predicted. Magical! Her handwriting has improved, she has gone up several reading levels at school, and our entire family life has calmed down. She has calmed down and finally feels like she can succeed. I am tearful with gratitude that you helped talk me through this and opened the door to so much happiness."

If a patient doesn't respond to one stimulant after an adequate dosing trial, it helps to try other stimulants as another may work. If none of them work, the next medicine to try is Strattera. It works on norepinephrine, not dopamine, takes several weeks rather than a few days to act, and is helpful throughout the twenty four hour span of the day. (The stimulants cause insomnia if taken too late in the day.) If Strattera is ineffective, a third tier medication called Intuniv may prove useful. It is especially useful for those who are very anxious or who have tics, which get worse on the stimulants and Strattera. Some patients do not respond to any medications, in which case the behavioral and nutritional approaches are the mainstay of treatment.

Elder Sommers did respond well to Adderall XR. He was finally able to concentrate when reading his scriptures and said that his mind stayed with his eyes as he read down the page. He also felt less bored as he and his companion knocked on doors, and he was able to follow the discussions and do his part without any problem. He also found it much easier to pay attention in conferences and during the three hours of church on Sunday. He did pay a price for his improvement, however. He became more serious and less playful on his medicine. He felt it was a price he was willing to pay to be a more effective missionary.

This led to a discussion about his goals in life. He didn't yet know what he wanted to do but had some interest in becoming a computer graphic designer so he could make new games. His active and creative mind would need a field of endeavor that engaged him fully. The choice of a career is extremely important for an ADHD person, and I told Elder Sommers to be sure to pick a field he enjoyed. That alone would help him pay attention.

He also discussed his desire to go to college and his fears that he would not do well. I told him that schooling for ADHD people is a different experience when they treat their condition with medication. They can pay attention better in lectures and find it easier to take notes without being distracted. They can read and retain what they have read. They don't procrastinate. They are less overwhelmed. I reminded him that he needed to do his work while his Adderall was in his system rather than waiting until the end of the day as he had in high school. I also reminded him that he needed to apply the organizational skills he had learned on his mission to manage the seemingly abundant free time he would have in college. Elder Sommers was bright and creative, so I encouraged him to go to college and apply his gifts.

As his mission neared its end, his thoughts turned to dating. He had dated in high school but had never had a long term girlfriend. An older brother had had trouble that he did not want to repeat. He told me that he thought he needed a wife who would "keep me in line," correct his ADHD behaviors and problems so he would be successful. This reminded me of his mother, worried about his success but expressing it with criticism and punishment. I told him that the world would give him plenty of criticism and correction, so it was nice to come home to someone who was patient and supportive, who could see the positive and help him grow.

Elder Sommers finished his mission and went to work to save money for school. He alternately worked for a semester for his uncle, who was a building contractor, and went to school for a semester. He was a much better student and eventually became a physical therapist. This field was a good choice for him because it allowed him to work with people and to move around during his work day. His warmth and humor contributed to his success.

## Chapter 6: Body Dysmorphic Disorder

*Glory be to God for dappled things--*
*For skies of couple-colour as a brinded cow;*
*For rose-moles all in stipple upon trout that swim;*
*Fresh-firecoal chestnut-falls; finches' wings;*
*Landscape plotted and pieced--fold, fallow, and plough;*
*And all trades, their gear and tackle and trim.*
*All things counter, original, spare, strange;*
*Whatever is fickle, freckled (who knows how?)*
*With swift, slow; sweet, sour; adazzle, dim;*
*He fathers-forth whose beauty is past change:*
*Praise him.*

--"Pied Beauty" by Gerard Manley Hopkins[xiii]

Good, I thought as I rounded the corner into the waiting room, my new patient is handsome. I will enjoy looking at him for the next nineteen months. He had dark brown hair, beautiful eyes, and a perfectly proportioned face, though it was subdued and sad looking. I invited Elder Johnson up to my office and asked how I could help him. He looked embarrassed as he confessed that his greatest problem was that he was so ugly. It tormented him every waking moment and made missionary work agonizingly difficult. He felt people turned away from him in disgust.

He said that after his morning shower, he would fix his hair and then redo it numerous times. On the street he would look at his reflection in store windows or car mirrors. At zone conferences he would excuse himself to go to the bathroom so he could look at himself in the mirror for awhile to check on his hair and assess his appearance. This also gave him a way to avoid contact with the sister missionaries. While he was reading the scriptures, knocking on doors, teaching discussions, or attending meetings, his mind was double tracking, thinking of his looks. It was exhausting and discouraging. He suffered from body dysmorphic disorder.

I asked him when this had started, and he told me it began in early adolescence, twelve or thirteen years old. What had led up to it? When he was ten and eleven, he started to fight a lot with his mother. He was oppositional to her; everything and anything became a battle, and he carried grudges about it all. When his father came home at night, my patient would complain to him, and the father would side with his son and argue with the mother. She angrily told Elder Johnson that if the marriage broke up, it would be his fault.

I wondered if Elder Johnson felt that he was ugly on the inside as a result of his arguments with his mother, and this became a fear that he was ugly on the outside His symptoms unfolded through his adolescence. His profound dissatisfaction focused on his face, especially his hair. He felt he never had a good hair day. Haircuts were fraught with anxiety. If he thought it was a bad haircut, it intensified his symptoms for weeks. He spent hours in front of the mirror looking at every tiny detail. He would put his face a few inches from the mirror, and at that distance every small blemish was magnified enormously. His complaints were that his face was round and fat, not chiseled, that he had extra skin under his chin, that his face was asymmetrical, that he did not like his hair, eyebrows, or eyes, that he hated his jaw line and profile, that he looked ugly from different angles, and that he looked bland and average.

He bought pictures of the handsomest male movie stars and compared each element of his face with theirs. Once he did not leave his room for a week while doing this. He mourned that he would never be as successful as Brad Pitt and felt envious that Brad Pitt's looks had handed him life on a silver platter. Since he believed that others measured a person's worth by his looks, he had no chance of succeeding. The odd thing was that Elder Johnson was handsome enough to be a movie star.

His parents became alarmed as they realized the distress their son was suffering. They reassured him that he was very good looking, but this only seemed to increase his craving for more reassurance. Mrs. Johnson enrolled him in modeling classes, and a prestigious store wanted to hire him as a model for the posters in their stores. Mrs. Johnson would buy clothes for her son which would help for a short while, but he would soon sink into his illness again. His father and mother did everything they could to help him overcome Body Dysmorphic Disorder, including taking him to a psychiatrist for psychotherapy and medication.

The *Diagnostic and Statistical Manual of Mental Disorders (Fifth Edition)*[xiv] lists the diagnostic criteria for Body Dysmorphic Disorder (BDD) as follows:

- Preoccupation with one or more perceived defects or flaws in physical appearance that are not observable or appear slight to others
- At some point during the course of the disorder, the individual has performed repetitive behaviors (e.g. mirror checking, excessive grooming, skin picking, reassurance seeking) or mental acts (e.g. comparing his or her appearance with that of others) in response to the appearance concerns
- The preoccupation causes clinically significant distress or impairment in social, occupational, or other important areas of functioning

The most common areas of dissatisfaction are skin, hair, and nose, but any body area can be the focus of concern. Common behaviors are comparing one's appearance with others, repeatedly checking perceived defects in the mirror (up to five hours per day), excessive grooming, camouflaging with makeup or hats, seeking reassurance, touching disliked areas to check them, or seeking cosmetic surgical procedures. There is a 2.4% prevalence in adults in the United States, but it may be more common because many people don't divulge their suffering even to a therapist unless directly asked.

The most common age of onset is twelve to thirteen years of age. BDD has been associated with high rates of childhood abuse and neglect. The presence is increased in first degree relatives of those with obsessive compulsive disorder. Rates of suicide and suicide attempts are high in those with BDD. Major depressive disorder is the most common comorbidity and is often secondary to the distress of BDD. Nearly all those with BDD have impaired psychosocial functioning because of their concerns about their appearance, and some never leave their house for years. MRI studies show that different areas of the brain light up when they look at themselves compared to healthy individuals. The areas that light up indicate that their view of themselves is focused on small details of their appearance rather than the whole, and their view is highly critical.

With this information in mind, I thought it was brave of Elder Johnson to come on his mission. I wanted so much to help him, to ease his suffering so he could enjoy his mission. Part of his treatment with me involved the use of medication. He was treated with major tranquilizers and antidepressants. The antidepressants were used for the BDD but also for a depression that was visible in his sad, haggard look and audible in his muted, cautious voice. These medicines were somewhat helpful, but much less so than in many other psychiatric disorders like unipolar depression, bipolar depression, or obsessive compulsive disorder.

Elder Johnson's mother loaned me a copy of the book *The Broken Mirror* by Katharine Phillips, M.D. Dr. Phillips was the national expert on BDD, and her book was literally a godsend. I read it and shared it with Elder Johnson. We began with the list of common cognitive errors. These include eleven elements: all or nothing (black or white) thinking, mind reading, fortune telling, thinking with our feelings, labeling, discounting the positive, negative filtering, personalization, overgeneralization, catastrophizing, and unfair comparisons. Elder Johnson had ten of these. We used the list throughout his work to remind him to challenge and restructure his thinking.

We also did mirror retraining. I told him that after his morning shower he could fix his hair once while looking at the foggy mirror and then had to leave the bathroom. We decided that he could check his hair twice more during the day rather than many times. He could look in the mirror from a normal distance, but was not allowed to get up two inches from the mirror to examine his face. In addition, he was not to buy magazines on P day that showed "The World's Handsomest Men" so that he could not compare his facial features with theirs in the mirror.

A challenging part of our work involved behavior experiments and the use of charts modeled on Dr. Phillip's suggestions. We would together decide upon a challenge on which he could work until the next session when he would report his results. Some of our choices were:

- Go into Sacrament meeting without checking in the mirror first. Look at three people and greet them with a smile.
- While going to the grocery store on P day, speak to two people in line at the checkout. If they were unresponsive, assume they were having a hard day instead of assuming they were repulsed by his ugliness.
- Make conversation with several of the sister missionaries at conferences instead of going into the bathroom to avoid them.

- Spend time at the end of his day with the other elders in the living room without checking his appearance in the mirror beforehand.
- Work on NOT comparing himself with a handsome companion.

Sometimes he would come in elated over his successes, but other times when he was more depressed he would not have tried. These setbacks were greeted with understanding combined with encouragement to keep trying.

Early in our work I made the mistake of reassuring Elder Johnson that he was indeed very handsome. I could see that he craved this but that it did no lasting good. It was actually counterproductive because it intensified his need and longing for it, so I stopped. He also worked on not asking others for reassurance during the week. He improved from asking many times per day to just twice a week.

We did have an ever increasing bond as we struggled with his suffering. I saw him weekly for fifty minute sessions that combined medication management with psychotherapy. It was difficult to sit with him during the early months of our work because his anxiety and depression were palpable, but gradually he became better. He began to smile more, to develop creative ways of working with the members to help them make referrals. After nine months of our work, he experienced two weeks of blissful freedom from his torment. He felt wonderful. It is hard to say how long this would have lasted, but he and his companion decided to intensify their work for a week. They pushed themselves extremely hard, fasting, forgoing any breaks, working throughout P day. The increased stress with attendant elevated cortisol levels caused a return of his symptoms.

Several years after his return home he went to see Dr. Katharine Phillips for a consultation. She called to ask me how we had accomplished that miraculous two weeks of freedom from his illness. She said that is unheard of in this condition. I shared my approach, using her book and charts, and listed the medications he had taken, but there were several elements in our work that I couldn't convey to her. One element was the strength of our relationship. We were a team, working hard together against his BDD. He told his parents he felt that our work was incredibly helpful to him, that I was his best friend and an angel sent to help him.

A second element was spiritual. I prayed fervently asking for help with our work and comfort for him. So did he. Elder Johnson wrote, "I wearied the Lord continually for his help and assistance. I made it a matter of prayer and did so with real intent, a sincere heart, and an abundance of faith that Christ would help me." Along with prayer, he listed work as a second factor that played a major role in his personal conversion. In spite of his suffering, he stayed on his mission and was obedient, faithful, and hard working. His decision to stay led to wonderful spiritual growth. He wrote, "I can remember the transfer that my mission changed. That my life changed. I, in a literal sense, was saved by Christ's atoning sacrifice. I experienced a mighty change of heart. I became converted. I now continually have that strong personal conversion to give me the strength and courage to fight against life's great storms and I no longer try to do so without the help of God." Elder Johnson was not the only missionary I treated who grew spiritually in the fashion he described, but he certainly had the toughest opposition on a daily basis.

I spoke with him recently, and he is still using the behavioral approach we learned from *The Broken Mirror*. He has been able to come off his medicine and is not depressed. He is a senior in college and has decided to become a clinical psychologist so that he can help others find relief from difficulties. He will bring a depth of compassion and wisdom to his work which he developed through his own suffering.

## Chapter 7: Asperger's Syndrome

*And at nine years of age, I had a life-changing revelation. I figured out how to talk to other children. I suddenly realized that when a kid said, "Look at my Tonka truck," he expected an answer that made sense in the context of what he had said.*

*Here were some things I might have said prior to this revelation in response to "Look at my Tonka truck."*
*a.) "I have a helicopter."*
*b.) "I want some cookies."*
*c.) "My mom is mad at me today."*
*d.) "I rode a horse at the fair."*

*I was so used to living inside my own world that I answered with whatever I had been thinking. If I was remembering riding a horse at the fair, it didn't matter if a kid came up to me and said, "Look at my truck!" or "My mom is in the hospital!" The other kid's words did not change the course of my thoughts. All of a sudden, I realized that the response the kid was looking for, the correct answer, was:*
*e.) "That's a neat truck! Can I hold it?"*

*Look Me in the Eye* by John Elder Robinson[xv]

Elder William Thomas sat in the waiting room full of patients, eyes on the floor, in his own world. I greeted him for our first session, and he rose to follow, avoiding my gaze and unresponsive to my greeting. He was tall and lanky and had to bend his head to enter my office. When he was settled on the couch, I asked him how I could help him, and he shared his painful story.

He had been in first grade when his only friend and he were playing on the playground. His friend decided to tie him up as part of their game, and William had a panic attack when he could not get free. Thereafter through sixth grade during recess he hid in a stack of tires where he felt safe. By middle school his isolation became unbearable, and he became clinically depressed. He was suicidal in his loneliness. As he entered the adolescent era, he intuitively knew he needed the companionship of his peers but this seemed an impossible accomplishment.

He turned his attention to turtles and became an expert in every facet of their world: their habitats, varieties, patterns, life cycles. His knowledge of them became encyclopedic. I looked at him and thought about turtles' ability to draw all parts of their bodies into their shells, into a safe space, like William hiding in his stack of tires on the playground. But turtles can't survive if they are permanently hiding.

William had a sister several years older who did have friends, and this kind sister allowed him to hang around with them, observing their interactions, learning how to relate to others. He had one date in high school, going to his junior prom. It was awkward and frightening, but he survived it.

His mission was a great challenge for him. It was all about relating to people, his greatest vulnerability. It was difficult to be with a companion all the time. He did not like small talk and was not interested in their lives. He didn't know what to say or how to connect when knocking on doors. He dreaded discussions because it felt so awkward to talk with strangers. He was alone in a crowd, so church meetings and mission conferences were a constant reminder of his isolation. He did not adapt well to change, so transfers were anxiety provoking. He could not feel the Holy Ghost, so bearing witness of the Gospel felt hollow. It all felt exquisitely painful and caused intense anxiety. He began to get depressed again and was referred to me for help. From his history I realized that he had

Asperger's syndrome because of the combination of social difficulties, lack of eye contact, dislike of small talk, encyclopedic knowledge of his area of interest, and heightened sense of fear.

Elder Thomas was difficult to treat. His companions had found it hard to relate to him and had complained to the mission president that he did not connect with investigators. It was equally challenging to connect with him in therapy. As he entered my office, my muscles would tighten in anticipation of the hour of tension ahead. He would settle stiffly on the couch and sit quietly until I would begin with the inevitable, "How are you? How are things going?" His mechanical response was invariably, "Fine." He still had twelve months to go on his mission when we started, so gradually as the months went by, I gleaned bits of information about his world. "Do you like your new companion?" I asked after a recent transfer. "He's O.K." "Is he a hard worker?" "Yes." "Is that O.K. with you?" "Yes, it's O.K."

Slowly by patient and persistent questioning, aided by information from the mission president, the ice began to thaw. The answers went from wooden, unrevealing statements to bits of shared information. After another transfer, I asked, "How is your new companion?" and was rewarded with the information that this companion talked constantly and loudly, assaulting my patient's very sensitive hearing. "That must be very tough," I said. "At least you are half way through this transfer. Could you tell the mission president about this so that you can be transferred to a quieter companion?" He looked startled. It had not occurred to him that he could make his life better. I reminded him that his auditory sensitivity was a part of his Asperger's syndrome and that his sensitivity to music, something I had recently learned about, was also an aspect of Asperger's for some people. "Would you give that gift up?" A faint smile crossed his somber face. His love of classical music had been his only solace in his isolation. I asked, "Do you talk with your companions about music?" "No," he answered. "I don't think any of them listen to classical music." "You never know until you ask. If would be a wonderful bond." Several transfers later he spontaneously reported that his new companion played the cello and knew all about classical music. He looked actually happy.

I knew that the hours we spent talking about his experiences and feelings were vital in helping him to learn to connect. He remained reserved in our sessions, but he became more expressive. The improvement carried over into his relationships with companions and his abilities as a missionary. I treated his depression and anxiety with an antidepressant. This relieved much of his suffering and helped him relax as he learned to connect more with others. When he finished his mission we had a final session, and as Elder Thomas left the office he did not shake my hand or thank me. Expressing gratitude is a social skill many Asperger's people do not possess. In his formality and emotional distance, he felt like ice.

In contrast, Elder Roger Field felt like fire. Everything about him was intense and passionate. He came to me because trusted friends told him to get treatment for his anxiety. He grew up in a family which moved around constantly. This made it difficult to sustain friendships, and he blamed this for his social difficulties. He moved at the start of eighth grade and felt that everyone in his new school was already in their social bubble. He was able to make friends with his scoutmaster's son, but the boy dropped him after three months. "He didn't want me in his social group." He was a social outcast all through high school and attributed this to his church membership and to his choice to belong to the marching band rather than running track. He went to a church college and had an awful experience. He felt that his rejection was because he had not yet served a mission. He had fewer than ten dates over these years, but not for lack of trying.

His mother was the "champion torch bearer" in supporting his self esteem. His father was also supportive, but at times they were in conflict. He provoked his father about not serving a mission for which his father punched him and kicked him out of the house. He then stayed at college and didn't come home so he could avoid the family.

Roger applied for a mission seven times and was rejected each time. A therapist at college wrote that he was a rebel and shouldn't go on a mission. Another therapist assessed him as very angry and lacking social skills. He said he couldn't stand Roger. In spite of these setbacks, Roger continued his efforts to go on a mission and was finally successful. I have never known another missionary who was so determined to go on a mission or was so persistent in overcoming the odds. It was admirable.

Once on his mission, Elder Field continued to have trouble. He had eleven companions in his first ten months. He had three emergency transfers away from companions who could not bear to be with him, but he had no idea why. He had been out on his mission for a year (counting the MTC) when I first met him. He wanted leadership opportunities and wondered why none came his way. He told me he considered himself a fine missionary because he gave love to people, but added that if they didn't accept it he quickly withdrew it.

Sessions with Elder Field were stressful because he was so emotionally intense, flaring up in anger over perceived injustices or misperceptions. "Dr. Payne, I went to district meeting, and the district leader gave the stupidest lesson. Why should he be the district leader? I could do so much better a job!" As he shared this, his face became red, his eyes bulged, and he clenched his fists. "I gave some of my ideas, some really good ideas, and he just ignored me like I was invisible. I hate this area. It is dead. The people in the ward are not friendly. They don't give us any leads. It's the worst area in the whole mission, and it's the second time I have had to be here."

"I'm sorry that you have not been put in leadership positions. I know you have a lot of strength and would be a good leader. Maybe people are intimidated by you because of your anger," I responded. "But my anger comes out when I say what I really feel. I won't be a fake. I say what I feel." I thought of the many Asperger patients I have known who prided themselves on their honesty and emotional bluntness. I answered, "Yes, you have that choice, but you suffer consequences for it. It costs you relationships and opportunities." He replied abruptly, "Well maybe I don't want those relationships anyway." "Elder Field, you are lonely. You want to go home and find someone to marry. It will help you if you moderate your anger and watch what you say."

Elder Field looked deflated, helpless. I realized that his anger made him feel powerful and without it he felt defenseless. I added, "We will work on other ways to help you feel in control in your life."

Considering his record of social difficulties, I wondered with Elder Field if he might have Asperger's syndrome. His area of special interest was baseball. He knew every statistic for each World Series and detailed statistics for his favorite teams and players. This is typical of the gifts of memory and knowledge that Asperger's people have. His temper was classically Asperger's. His level of stress in every area of his life matched as well. His lack of empathy was striking. A friend of mine told me that when Elder Field was serving in our ward she had invited him and his companion to dinner along with a handicapped soldier. The soldier had stepped on a land mine in Afghanistan. His leg was blown off, and he sustained multiple internal injuries. He was talking about his physical therapy with his artificial leg while they were all at dinner and shared with pride that he had run a twenty minute mile. Elder Field responded, "A twenty minute mile! I ran better than that in fourth grade. That's nothing to brag about." The young children in the family pounced on him and exclaimed, "But with one leg!" He then realized his faux pas and graciously praised the soldier for serving his country.

As I discussed the symptoms of Asperger's, Elder Field denied that he had any of them. He said that he had connected with many kinds of investigators and baptized them, so he must have social skills. He did not make the connection between my diagnosis and his social difficulties in multiple settings. This response was unusual. When I told other people about the diagnosis, they typically responded with relief to finally understand why they were as they were. I explained that there were many gifts as part of Asperger's syndrome: the logical, precise mind, the vast array of knowledge in their area of interest, their pleasure in sharing this knowledge, the gifts that often accompanied their heightened senses. Patients were also relieved to understand that those with Asperger's have a heightened response to stress. Life is genuinely more stressful for them than for most other people, but they persevere anyway.

Elder Field may have needed to reject my diagnosis because he didn't want to think there was anything "wrong" with him. He was defensive because of the many emotional blows he had received. He did accept the use of an antidepressant for depression and a mood stabilizer for temper. We continued to work together until he finished his mission. He was allowed to go home a little early because his mission president had run out of people who would be his companion, but he was rightly assured that he had served a full and honorable mission. I felt proud of him. He endured to the end and gave all he could. He was the first in his family to serve a mission for many generations and set a good example for the generations to follow.

Both of these elders are examples of Asperger's syndrome. As a pair they demonstrate that a diagnosis is but a part of a unique personality. No two people with any given diagnosis are just alike. I use this diagnosis but also note that it is no longer listed as a diagnosis in the Diagnostic and Statistical Manual of Mental Disorders V. It has been subsumed under the broader category of Autistic spectrum disorders. This is unfortunate since there are great differences between Autism and Asperger's syndrome. Autistic people are often severely impaired; about fifty percent of them are unable to speak, are intellectually impaired, and cannot live on their own as adults. Those with Asperger's syndrome, on the other hand, usually live normal lives. It is a broad spectrum, but most have careers and many marry and have children. Much of the literature regarding Asperger's gives examples from the most impaired end of the spectrum and ignores the more subtle presentations.

When the new DSM V was released at the American Psychiatric Association meetings in May, 2013, I attended an all day seminar regarding the new manual. When the presenters discussed the changes in the Autistic spectrum section they noted that this change had to do with access to funding for people with these disorders, but that because Asperger's syndrome as a diagnosis has been in such general usage and is so useful, it will continue to be available as a diagnosis.

I have included my own list of symptoms of Asperger's syndrome based on twenty years of treatment and extensive learning through reading the psychiatric literature and attending professional courses:

- Logical, precise mind
- Areas of special interest--the person knows a great deal about these areas and often enjoys talking at others about their knowledge, though sometimes missing the social cue that others have heard enough and would like to change the subject. They make excellent teachers.
- Screen time is a preferred way to spend time. It may be movies, news, sports, genealogy, computer games, browsing the web, or social media. When Asperger's people are in front of their preferred screen, they generally feel peaceful.
- Attention Deficit Hyperactivity Disorder is frequently present.

- Obsessive compulsive disorder is also frequently present.
- May have a strong temper with tantrums in childhood. May say unkind things without understanding how hurtful they are.
- Gross and fine motor coordination may be impaired. May have an unusual pencil grasp.
- Heightened sensitivity to stress
- Heightened senses
    - Visual: observant, photographic memory, excellent photographer
    - Auditory: cannot screen out ancillary sounds. Musically gifted. May have perfect pitch. May have synesthesia (e.g. may see a color or feel an emotion in connection with a certain musical note)
    - Olfactory: may be able to smell far more sensitively than others (e.g. a patient bragged that she could tell when milk was going sour days before anyone else in the family. Another liked to smell all her birthday presents before she opened them to see if any of them had a pleasant scent.)
    - Tactile: likes deep pressure, not light touch. May be bothered by clothing that doesn't feel just right.
    - Gustatory: may be a picky eater. May be able to assess seasonings with extraordinary precision. May become a fine chef.
    - Temperature: May be indifferent to cold
    - Pain: May have a heightened or lower threshold of pain
    - Fear: May have a heightened sense of fear.

- Interpersonal difficulties
    - Limited friendships
    - Discomfort in unstructured social settings, dislike of small talk
    - Can function well in a prescribed role at work or church
    - Trouble expressing and/or understanding feelings
    - Often have a pattern of parallel lives in their marriages with each spouse going about their business with little interaction. They may have separate checking accounts, go on separate vacations, or go to different restaurants when they go out to dinner.
- A sense of being different than other people but not knowing why. May get feedback from others saying, "You're weird!"
- Attraction to animals, who are simpler to relate to than people. Sometimes they have an extensive knowledge about dogs or penguins or whales, etc.

People do not have to have every characteristic on the list to have Asperger's syndrome, but they will have a number of these traits.

As with any diagnosis, not all of these symptoms need to be present to make the diagnosis, but when enough of them are present, there is no other explanation for the constellation of symptoms. It is also, as I have mentioned, a spectrum ranging from mild to severe. The percentage of Asperger's syndrome is uncertain. Various studies indicate rates ranging from one case in two hundred and fifty to one in ten thousand. Studies need to be performed with widely accepted criteria, a proper screening instrument, and acknowledgement of the broad spectrum of presentation.

In all studies it is listed as a disorder more common in males, with a ratio of 4:1 found in some studies. There was recently an article in the *Journal of the American Academy of Child and Adolescent Psychiatry* indicating that Asperger's syndrome is modified in females compared to males because females are by nature more attuned to relationships than males. They often have gifts that soften the social difficulties inherent in this condition.

There are differences at both macroscopic and microscopic levels in the brains of those with this syndrome. These differences develop while the fetus is forming and are in place at birth.

Treatment of Asperger's syndrome best begins in childhood by involving children in organized group activities like scouting, sports teams, chess clubs, and summer camps. It is also helpful to invite other children over to play. A perceptive mother can offer feedback and suggestions to improve the quality of the interaction. It is useful to involve the child in play therapy with an experienced child psychiatrist who can help facilitate communication, model empathy, and work with parents to understand their child. It is also useful to offer group therapy with peers if this is available. If people learn that they have Asperger's syndrome when they are older, it is still useful to be involved in social activities, individual or group therapy.

Going on a mission can be a rich experience for those with Asperger's syndrome because of the intense social exposure afforded by the nature of a mission. It is a theater of structured interaction. I have watched missionaries with this diagnosis make great strides when they experience a patient and loving companion.

There is one diagnostic combination that is particularly difficult: the combination of Asperger's syndrome and bipolar disorder. In all my years of practice, these patients have been the most impaired. I have treated three of them for over twenty years each and know firsthand how much they suffer in life. Very few of the missionaries I have treated have gone home early from their missions, eight out of many hundreds, and half of them were bipolar and Asperger's. The remainder were bipolar or schizophrenic and went home in the midst of a psychotic break. They were suffering too intensely to remain on their mission.

There is a role for medications in the treatment of Asperger's syndrome. All those with this condition have some degree of Attention Deficit Hyperactivity Disorder, so stimulant medication can be very helpful. If they develop a depression, antidepressants treat it. Antidepressants also help lessen anxiety in social situations; some of my Asperger's patients have been able to date and marry because they were so much better socially on antidepressants. For those with terrible tempers, mood stabilizers have helped to lessen the intensity and duration of their outbursts. These medicines have also eliminated the physical aggression that accompanied their temper outbursts. Some of my patients have punched holes in walls, broken glass furniture, repeatedly thrown and broken cell phones, or attacked people. It is important to stop these behaviors if they plan to succeed in life.

The omega three fatty acids are also helpful for Asperger's syndrome and should be used throughout life. They are of course useful in maintaining mood but also help diminish aggression.

A further difficulty for missionaries with Asperger's syndrome is that they may not be able to feel the Holy Ghost, which communicates through subtle feelings. The logical and precise manner of thinking that is a hallmark of Asperger's runs on a different track. I have known members with this syndrome who have been active in the Church for many years who said they live the Gospel so that, in case it is true, they will be on the right side. I admire these members who devote their lives to the Gospel without the sustaining, life-nourishing experiences that are given by the Holy Ghost. I have treated Mormon adolescents with Asperger's syndrome who did not go on missions or who left the Church because they could not feel its truth. Knowing them has increased my appreciation for those missionaries with Asperger's who did choose to come on a mission and share the Gospel, even when they could not feel the comforting presence of the Holy Ghost.

## Chapter 8: Mission Impossible

*Turning and turning in the widening gyre*
*The falcon cannot hear the falconer;*
*Things fall apart; the centre cannot hold;*
*Mere anarchy is loosed upon the world,*
*The blood -dimmed tide is loosed, and everywhere*
*The ceremony of innocence is drowned;*
*The best lack all conviction while the worst*
*Are full of passionate intensity.*

--"The Second Coming" by William Butler Yeats[xvi]

From time to time I was called to help missionaries who had been sent home early from other missions. They were really ill. For example, Elder Mark DuBois became a senior companion to a very unmotivated junior companion and felt like an utter failure when he could not get him going. Mark became depressed, withdrawn, dysfunctional, and finally mute. The mission doctor thought he might be schizophrenic and placed him on antipsychotic medication. The doctor accompanied him on the plane to get him safely home.

Within a few days of his arrival home, his mother brought Mark to my office. I greeted them in the waiting room and invited them upstairs. Kathryn DuBois was warm, pleasant, and eager to help her son. He sat in the waiting room with downcast eyes. His face was handsome, narrow, with beautiful brown hair that arched over his temples, but his good looks were muted by the stamp of pain and fear on his face. He rose slowly and accompanied his mother, who came up with him to assist us since Mark remained almost mute. After they were settled side by side on the couch, I asked Mark what had happened on his mission. After a long pause, with great effort and very slowly, he answered, "I came home." This exhausted him and he sat silently. His mother waited quietly, respectful of her son's autonomy, but I cast a glance of appeal to her. She picked up the slender thread of conversation. "Mark is not usually like this. He has always been quiet, but he is usually much happier. He has always really been into his own thoughts." She added that he was very upset that he was sent home from his mission. It was not his choice, and he wanted to go back as soon as possible.

As months passed, Mark slowly came alive. His mother continued to sit in on every other session for the first year. It was difficult for him to put his thoughts into words, so everything happened in slow motion. My mind moved quickly, and I had to still my thoughts as I waited patiently for him to share something. Each sentence from him was a gift. One day he brought a journal to show me. "What do you write in it?" I asked. At that point in our work he was able to answer fully. He said, "I write down my creative ideas that would make life better for people." "How would you do that?" I asked. "I love superheroes. I want to be one of them, to help people." The next session he brought me a DVD of Disney's Hercules. It was a sure sign that he was getting better, I thought, that he had brought me this present. He asked me in the next session if I had watched it. "I haven't had time to watch it yet, but I will by the time you come again." I did watch it and was prepared to discuss it with him, but he didn't want to discuss it. In his matter-of-fact tone, he said, "It was a loan, not a gift." I was embarrassed by the misunderstanding and returned it the following session.

This exchange opened the way for us to explore his wish to be a superhero. I asked, "Are there people you have been able to help?" "Not really. Not yet. I did like a girl once. I asked her out, but she was already engaged. So I tried to help her by giving her a wedding gift. It was decorated with charms that stood for love, cooperation, and so on, to help her have a happy marriage."

As I watched Mark's handsome face, I thought of his wish to be a hero. He emphasized that he had become dysfunctional on his mission not because of his unmotivated junior companion, but because of his own failure to adequately lead that companion. In other words, he had failed to be a hero in his own eyes. But to me he *was* a hero. He was so introverted and yet he had bravely gone on his mission, and when he had trouble and had to come home, he wanted nothing more than to go back again.

I was treating Mark for severe depression and attributed his slowness of thought and speech to that. He went to bed around 2 AM and slept for ten or twelve hours, but his mother had the same pattern of sleep. I also thought his lack of motivation was due to depression. I had seen this many times and had also seen it resolve as the depression lifted. I treated him with several antidepressants, increasing the doses gradually, but he showed little improvement. He did become more able to carry on a conversation, but my efforts to help him engage in life bore no fruit.

Although Mark did not have any hallucinations or delusions, I began to reconsider my diagnosis. I remembered the diagnosis given him by the mission doctor: schizophrenia. Elements that favored this diagnosis were mistrust of others on the mission, muteness, and abnormal sleep. Added to these were the slowness of his recovery in spite of treatment and his utter lack of motivation to get a job, go to school, or socialize.

Schizophrenia is defined in the *Diagnostic and Statistical Manual of Mental Disorders, Fifth Edition*[xvii], as follows:

- Positive symptoms
  - Delusions (distortions in thought content, like the thought that the radio is beaming signals from the CIA intended to control one's mind)
  - Hallucinations (hearing, seeing, tasting, feeling, or smelling things that do not really exist--most

frequently hearing voices as if they came from the outside world)
- Disorganized speech and behavior (derailment, incoherence, or mutism)

- Grossly disorganized or catatonic behavior (remaining in one position for hours)

- Negative symptoms
    - Losing interest in everyday activities such as bathing, grooming, or getting dressed.
    - Feeling out of touch with other people, family, or friends
    - Lack of emotion (apathy)
    - Having inappropriate feelings in certain situations (like laughing when someone has died)
    - Having less ability to experience pleasure
    - Reduced drive to pursue goal directed behavior (avolition)

People with schizophrenia may also develop depression, anxiety disorders like panic attacks, and cognitive disorders. Schizophrenia is a heterogeneous clinical syndrome, that is, it has many different clinical forms. A recent study reviewed in *Psychiatric News* stated that there are eight different genomic types of schizophrenia which present with different clinical syndromes. At least two positive symptoms must be present for a month or longer. Disorganized and negative symptoms may also be present. In addition, the level of functioning in work, interpersonal relations, and self care is far below that shown before the illness began. There may be hostility and aggression.

Schizophrenia affects one percent of the population worldwide. Males usually become ill in the late teens or early twenties, but females usually are well until their late twenties or thirties because of the protective effect of estrogen. Females are therefore more likely to marry, have children, and have finished their education before the illness strikes.

Some schizophrenics have periodic episodes of psychosis and seem normal between episodes. Signs of relapse include:

- Disturbed sleep patterns
- Fearful or tense feelings
- Difficulty concentrating
- Agitation and irritability
- Difficulty with simple, everyday tasks
- Excessive tiredness and lack of energy
- Loss of interest in activities
- Confusion and disordered thinking
- Reappearance or worsening of psychotic symptoms, such as delusions or hallucinations.

If they are in treatment, relapse is often because they have stopped taking their medication. This frequently happens because they don't think they need it anymore, don't like the side effects, or think it is poisoning them. Actually, the antipsychotics now available for the treatment of psychotic conditions are indispensable in the stabilization of the illness and the prevention of long term damage to the brain. Other patients show a slowly progressive downhill course which impairs their executive functioning and makes it very difficult to work or live independently.

Schizophrenics have problems with memory, language usage, organization, control of impulses, slowness in processing information, and problems with concentration. They may also misread the intentions and feelings of those around them. These problems are often present continuously even for those who are only intermittently psychotic.

*The Diagnostic and Statistical Manual, Fifth Edition*[xviii], states: "Psychotic symptoms tend to diminish over the life course...Negative symptoms are more closely related to prognosis than are positive symptoms and tend to be the most persistent. Schizophrenia is associated with significant social and occupational dysfunction. Making educational progress and maintaining employment are frequently impaired by avolition (lack of motivation) or other disorder manifestations, even when the cognitive skills are sufficient for the tasks at hand. Most individuals are employed at a lower level than their parents, and most, particularly men, do not marry or have limited social contacts outside their family."

When Mark came into treatment, he was suffering from depression, and the underlying schizophrenia was not obvious to me. As it came into focus, it explained the glacial progress. No wonder he resisted my efforts to help him reintegrate. I tried to treat him with several antipsychotic medications, but he was very sedated and didn't like them. Medication is the key to managing this illness and deserves many trials to find the best antipsychotic.

At this point I retired, and Mark began to work with my replacement. Months later his mother reported to me that he had stopped showering, shaving or attending to his clothing. His beautiful hair now hung in long and greasy strands. He was becoming increasingly angry and aggressive, was sleeping longer, and was starting to think of his parents as the enemy. She was frightened for her son. I could no longer give her medical advice since I had retired, but I consulted with my replacement who agreed with the diagnosis of schizophrenia, ever more apparent. She referred him to several clinics where he and his family would have a whole team to meet their needs. With this diagnosis it was clear that Mark would not be able to return to his mission.

Most people do not go back if they have come home early from a mission. Once home, their task is to build a life as an adult. It is also their task to mourn the loss of their mission. It is a loss tinged with shame, so the task of mourning becomes more complicated. It calls for the balm of forgiveness of one's supposed failure. This is more easily achieved if they remember that they were suffering too much to remain. If they could have finished, they would have.

When a missionary comes home early, he or she needs to be met with kindness, thoughtfulness, and support from members of his or her ward. There is no room for jokes, criticism, or gossip. Those in the ward can help the returned missionary to heal by treating him like a normal person and including him in activities.

The response of priesthood leaders is also of vital importance. I knew a missionary who had taken ADHD medication all his life. He stopped it when he went to the MTC and was soon overwhelmed. Once on his mission he became depressed, and at his eight month mark he mentioned to his companion that he wouldn't mind being hit by a truck. When this was reported to the mission president, he was quickly sent home. He and his family were devastated. I was sad to learn of the circumstances because depression is treatable. With proper psychiatric help for both depression and ADHD, he could have finished his mission.

The family was also hurt and upset that the mission president did not follow up with this elder. Although he had sent him home for being suicidal, he showed no further interest in him. I know mission presidents are incredibly busy, but it is good to remember not just the 99, but the one sheep who is lost. The stake president also showed a lackluster response, so the family felt abandoned by their priesthood leaders and continue to harbor feelings of bitterness and shame to this day.

In contrast, another missionary who was sent home early was treated with great kindness by his ward members. When he came to church that first Sunday, members of the ward said only,

"We're glad you're home. It's good to see you." The stake president told his parents to call him as soon as he got home, even if it was very late, because he wanted to meet with the returning elder. He continued to meet with him frequently. The Bishop also supported him with several interviews conducted with unconditional acceptance. He was asked to help with service projects, taken out to breakfast, and invited to go on splits with the missionaries. A member of the ward arranged for him to get a job. This elder was able to move on much more successfully.

Let me give another example. Sarah Benson called about her son Jim and asked if I could see him for a few months to help him get ready for his mission. My schedule was always full, but I thought I could make room for someone for a few months. Jim Benson arrived for his session, and as I greeted him, I thought, "What a kind face he has." He was tall and lean with brown hair, round brown eyes, and a shy smile. He had been a difficult child, the fourth of five children. Although he was a sweet boy, he had "unbelievable temper tantrums" including head banging which began in infancy. Irritability was a constant problem. He was shy, anxious, a very private person, and couldn't do the give and take of friendships. He was inflexible and needed great consistency in his routines. He had some learning disabilities. He was in the 95th percentile for math but only the 7th percentile for language. He also had a poor memory. So in spite of his excellent intelligence, school was frustrating for him. Jim's mother commented that his life was a series of failures. In high school he became depressed. He went to a child and adolescent psychiatrist who treated the depression, and he did well until he went off to college. He lived in a dorm with roommates, didn't take his medicine, and became depressed again. Jim failed his first semester and felt that his whole life was a miserable failure. He and his family decided to limit his academic hours to twelve per semester. His mother resumed her management of his medicine. He was then able to get a B average in his major, computer science.

It was at this point that Sarah Benson called me regarding her son. He was interested in going on a mission, and the parents wanted to know if there were accommodations that might help him. They also asked me to help prepare him psychologically for a mission.

He was still seeing the psychiatrist who had helped him with his adolescent depression. She was treating him with an antidepressant. Based on his history of irritability, tantrums, and dysphoria (unhappiness) throughout childhood, combined with his two depressions, I made the diagnosis of bipolar type II disorder. I assumed his care and treated him with bipolar medications for the next eleven years until my retirement. My diagnosis proved to be accurate. His mood fluctuated, requiring ongoing therapy and juggling of medications to keep it steady.

To get Jim ready for his mission, I collaborated with his bishop and stake president. Jim had a part time job, and his stake president wanted him to increase his work hours which would put him under maximal stress. That would give some idea of whether he could manage a mission. He also took over the management of his medication, a necessity for his mission. Jim was steady. He handled the stress extremely well and was able to oversee his medication. Two years after we had begun our work, I wrote a letter to his stake president that Jim was ready to serve a mission. He wanted to go to a foreign country, but I specified that he needed to remain in the United States where he could work with a psychiatrist in the mission field. I also asked that his mission president choose companions who could be patient and flexible with him.

Elder Jim Benson did well in the MTC, but after a short time in the mission field he felt very stressed, began to say strange things, and to act more aggressively. When the mission president decided to send him home, Elder Benson seemed relieved and was peacefully packing to go home when the mission doctor arrived to take him to the mission office. He wanted to come home to get his medication adjusted, and he knew he "was never going to get it right in the mission field." His mission president was supportive, reassuring him that he would be able to return to normal functioning with further professional help. All concerned agreed that the mission was too stressful for him. As mentioned in the chapter on bipolar disorder, stress is a major cause of destabilization in bipolar disorder. Cortisol levels elevated over time do no favors to any brain, especially that of a bipolar person.

When Jim Benson returned home, we resumed our work. He began, "I dread going to church because people know that I've come home early. Some come up and ask me point blank why I'm home too soon." "What do you say?" "I tell them I couldn't hack it!" He looked sad and ashamed. I responded, "People are curious, and I'm sure a lot of them are concerned. You grew up in that ward, and many of those people were your teachers and leaders, right?" He nodded his assent. "You are interpreting their interest as judgment and reproach. You are afraid of whispers behind your back. Maybe you could reframe it and experience their questions as concern." He burst out, "Well, then, what am I supposed to say?" I said, "Tell them it's a medical reason." "And if they keep asking?" His shoulders slumped, imagining this. "Then how about 'It's personal,' and that's the end of it." "But I feel like a failure again." "Wait a minute," I said. "You were worthy to go on a mission. In our crazy adolescent culture, that is wonderful. You went to the MTC and learned how to be a missionary, and then you went to the mission field to apply those skills. Now you can continue to do missionary work throughout your life."

Jim returned to college. He got a degree in computer science and then a job in his field. He became his boss's right hand man. He remained active in the church with callings that entailed much responsibility. He began to date, anxiously at first and then with increasing confidence. As mentioned, we worked hard to keep his mood steady.

Along the way it became apparent that Jim also had Asperger's syndrome. There is an overlap between the childhood symptoms of Asperger's and bipolar disorder. In both conditions the children are irritable and throw huge tantrums. The clues in Jim's history that pointed to Asperger's syndrome included his shyness, his interpersonal difficulties with roommates in college and missionary companions, and his great anxiety and initial awkwardness in dating. He also had wonderful musical ability that can be part of the sensory gifts of Asperger's. As mentioned in the chapter on Asperger's syndrome, people with this condition are more sensitive to stress. They also don't like change; his difficulty going off to college and then on his mission are understandable looked at from this perspective. In addition, his father, brother, and sister also had Asperger's syndrome. The combination of bipolar disorder and Asperger's syndrome makes it difficult to serve a mission.

There was a third factor in Jim's array of problems. After his return from his mission, Jim was diagnosed with chronic Lyme disease. He was treated by a local infectious disease doctor for several years. She prescribed high doses of antibiotics for prolonged periods of time. This is a controversial treatment, and many doctors in our area spoke against her methods, but for Jim Benson it worked wonders. To my surprise, his slowness of speech and memory problems resolved, and he became much more successful at his job and in his social life. Lyme disease affects the brain as well as many other parts of the body. People are complicated, and all aspects of their physical and mental health need to be taken into account.

I have never seen a missionary come home early for a superficial reason. I am sad for them, but I know how relieved most of them are. Throughout this book I have referred to the spiritual growth that comes from serving a mission. It is important to continue that growth after coming home, whether the missionary comes home after one month or twenty-four months. There are many missionaries who return and become inactive. But both Elder

DuBois and Elder Benson have remained active in the Church. Continued involvement in the Church leads to spiritual growth over time as our spirits soften and become more loving, obedient, and forgiving. This growth is not a competition--the pace is personal.

I am reminded of the book by John Groberg, "In the Eye of the Storm."[xix] The book is a record of his mission to Tonga, and during his mission he lived through a raging hurricane that stripped his island of food. At the four week marker a supply ship failed to arrive, and after nine weeks the people on the island were slowly starving and dying. Elder Groberg stopped moving around and sat still on the ground. He began to ponder the deeper realities of life and our role in the cosmos. He shared two ideas that have bearing on the problem of returning early from a mission.

1. The only thing that is important is your standing in the sight of your Father in Heaven. If that is as it should be, nothing else matters. If that is not as it should be, nothing else counts. If you die, you die, and it doesn't matter so long as you've done what is right, and the only thing that really matters is your standing in God's sight. When you feel God's love and have the confidence and assurance that He is there, then other things aren't important. You understand that what we're doing down here on earth all revolves around learning to love and serve God and our fellowman.

2. When we begin to understand the relationship of opposition to growth and start to sense the type of growth God has designed for us and is trying to help us achieve, we tend to give thanks rather than complain about obstacles to overcome. People unchallenged are largely people undeveloped, be it physically, emotionally, or spiritually.

Viewed in this context, closing the chapter of missionary service sooner rather than later is not a disaster but opens a new chapter for growth. Some people walk the path of life with long strides while others take short steps. The important question is: In which direction are you heading?

## Chapter 9: Gifts of the Spirit

*The Lord bless thee, and keep thee:*
*The Lord make his face shine upon thee, and be gracious unto thee:*
*The Lord lift up his countenance upon thee, and give thee peace.*

Numbers 6: 24-26

I have mentioned throughout these chapters that missionaries grow spiritually on their missions and have spiritual experiences and insights that aid this process. I have included some stories from family and friends to give examples of this process. These stories suggest that the core of missionary experience lies in developing and strengthening a relationship with each member of the Godhead. The fruit of this is a gradual softening of the spirit with the development of humility, patience, and love. These qualities make it easier to endure well to the end, whether it be the end of a mission, a difficult period of life, or life itself.

### Russell Armstrong

Brother Armstrong served in the South African mission. His second companion was the hardest experience of his mission. The companion was "edgy," aggressive, and entitled. His attitude was, "If you're not going to give it to me, I will take it." He felt he was special and that the rules didn't apply to him. (This is a good encapsulation of a narcissistic personality disorder.) They were together for three months. During that time Elder Armstrong felt very isolated and wasn't sure how he should react. His companion was emotionally abusive with the potential for physical assault, so Elder Armstrong was worried that he would turn on him. Once they were knocking on doors and came to a home with a vicious dog. The dog bit Elder

Armstrong, whose edgy companion revealed that he had a gun in their apartment and wanted to shoot the dog. It was all Elder Armstrong could do to dissuade him. After one more episode, this missionary was sent home early.

I asked Brother Armstrong how he had endured this experience. He had said that he had internalized his father's voice. His father had been a mission president and a stake president and had prepared him "to expect chaos." He also taught him to represent their family name and the Church proudly, so he knew how to behave well in the most adverse circumstances. His mission president was like a second father. He was supportive of all the missionaries and especially of Elder Armstrong since he was a friend of his father.

The third father to whom he turned for support and guidance was Heavenly Father. Elder Armstrong felt competent on his mission, but beginning with his frightening companion, he became less self-reliant and ever more reliant on the Lord. He took problems to the Lord in prayer and discussed them. His increasing mastery of the scriptures helped him work through difficult times as well. He said that the Savior became his confidant and best friend.

When his mission ended, he was released by his mission president because he had come from a district without a stake president whose duty it is to release returned missionaries. The other missionaries were all going to be released after they got home. It was difficult knowing that all the other elders would have the protective mantle of a mission during their homeward journey, while he would not. He began the journey home and was beset by doubts, fearing that he had not accomplished all that he wanted on his mission. He was sitting next to a pretty girl on the plane. He began to think of the temptations and challenges he would be facing back in the world. He felt steadily worse and decided to spend the whole flight in prayer. He then had the most profound spiritual experience of his life. He felt loved beyond measure by his Father. His doubts and fears melted away and were replaced by profound peace. His mission experience strengthened him for the rest of his life.

**Steve Morgan**

Elder Steve Morgan served in the Washington, DC, North mission. He had been on his mission only a short time when he and his companion began teaching Margoe and Robert Christensen. They had found the Christensens while knocking on doors. Margoe was a joy to teach, but her husband was more difficult. He smoked cigarettes, and it was hard to give them up. They knew they needed to teach them together, so in preparation they spent a day in prayer and fasting. That evening they took Brother Wilson, an older man from their ward, with them. Imagine their disappointment when Margoe answered the door and told them that her five month old baby daughter was very sick, so it was not a good night for the lesson. They could hear the baby screaming in the background. She had not slept all day and had a fever. Brother Wilson asked, "Have the missionaries taught you about priesthood blessings?" "No, not yet," Margoe answered. Brother Wilson explained what he meant, and Margoe and Robert both thought it sounded like an excellent idea. Elder Morgan anointed the infant as she screamed hysterically, but as soon as Brother Wilson began the blessing she stopped crying and fell asleep. She had no return of her illness. As they left, Robert handed Elder Morgan his cigarettes. Both joined the church.

Elder Morgan had come to the Washington DC North mission with seven other elders from the MTC. One had gone home early, but the remaining group had stayed close throughout the mission. When their mission came to a close, they would all spend the last forty-eight hours together in the mission president's home. They would go to the temple, have a wonderful home cooked meal, and meet with the mission president for three and a half hours to prepare for the next phase of life. They would have a testimony meeting. As he anticipated these events, he expected tears, sadness at the parting, regrets. He was surprised to find instead that the feelings were all positive. All seven had been obedient and had served good, faithful missions. They had finished well. They were looking forward, not back. They felt peaceful and were filled with joy to be going home honorably.

**Roger Morgan**

Elder Roger Morgan served in the Lansing, Michigan mission. He summarized the spiritual progress of his mission with the following four points:

1.) We are all in pursuit of happiness. Satan takes the truth about how to achieve happiness and twists it, confusing people and making them think that happiness comes from money, fame, or popularity.
2.) The uniform message from prophets is that we will be happy if we obey the commandments.
3.) How do we prioritize obedience? Jesus Christ told us the two greatest commandments were to love God and love our fellow men.
4.) How do we develop this love?

Elder Morgan learned on his mission that the key to love is service. On his mission, he had no time for himself, but was always serving others. He mentioned King Benjamin's address in Mosiah 2: 17, "And behold, I tell you these things that ye may learn wisdom; that ye may learn that when ye are in the service of your fellow beings, ye are only in the service of your God." So as we increase in love for others through service, we thereby increase our love for God.

**Brian Morgan**

Elder Brian Morgan served his mission in Brazil. He had studied Portuguese in the MTC, but once in Brazil, he found he couldn't understand anyone. He found that if he relied on the Holy Ghost to convey the essence of people's communications he could understand. He continued to refine his ability to feel the Holy Ghost and be led by it throughout his mission.

He and his companion taught a family, bringing the Holy Ghost with them for each discussion. The family was baptized and confirmed, gaining the permanent companionship of the Holy Ghost for themselves. The missionaries went to their home to visit them soon afterward, and when they opened their door, Elder Morgan felt the Holy Ghost come flowing outward from their home. They no longer needed the elders to bring it to them. Brian Morgan added that he maintained his sensitivity to the Holy Ghost, and it blesses his life daily.

**Eric Morgan**

Elder Eric Morgan served his mission in Guatemala. He said the most important lesson he learned on his mission is the manner in which the Holy Ghost speaks to us. He and his companion met a Catholic priest named Herman Diaz who was rising in the ranks of the Catholic church and had his heart set on becoming a cardinal. He had dealt with Mormon missionaries before and loved to have a good battle with them. He was disappointed that Elder Morgan and his companion were not fighters. After four visits, the elders told him they wouldn't come back anymore, but left him a Book of Mormon. They told him to pray about its truth. He read it in two days, then left his house and ran to find the missionaries. He said he was ready for baptism. After he joined the Church, he became the best missionary.

Months later, he and his companion planned a missionary night that was going to be fantastic, but one by one their appointments fell through. They looked at each other in bewilderment, wondering what to do with their evening. They decided to go visit Brother Diaz. When they arrived at his home and knocked on the door, he flung it open and without even looking at them exclaimed, "Elders, what took you so long? We have been praying that you would come, and finally you have." He had a young woman there, an investigator, whom they taught. She was baptized and brought her whole family into the church as well.

Elder Morgan spent his last ten months in a small town. The branch had only fifteen members, and those who held the priesthood were in short supply. He was made branch president. As a twenty year old with little experience in life, he found the call overwhelming. As he counseled couples about their problems, he tried to use his parents' excellent marriage as a model. Many of the couples were not married because the Guatemalan government had passed laws making it prohibitively expensive to marry. So people pretended to be married and had children. One couple with whom he worked especially troubled him. The man was somewhat abusive to the woman, the mother of his four children. She wanted to be baptized but had to either marry this man or leave him before she could become a member of the Church. She asked Elder Morgan his opinion. He personally felt that she should leave him, but when he opened his mouth to counsel her, these were the words that came out, "Sister, he loves you. It is not ideal, but no marriage is. He is the father of your children." It was an answer from Father in Heaven. He knew he was just the conduit. As branch president, he performed the marriage, and the next day she was baptized. He went back years later to visit his mission, and the couple was still happily married.

Elder Morgan felt that his mission brought him ever closer to the Holy Ghost and more reliant on the Lord.

**David Clayton**

"Early in my mission I had a companion who was not as eager as I was to be out tracting among the people or to obey the mission guidelines as I was. It was frustrating for me as a young missionary who wanted to work longer hours, get up and study on time, leave the house on time...One afternoon, lunch break turned into nap time and I was troubled, not knowing what to do to get out the door. I was praying in the other room, asking for help when my companion sprang out of his bed and said he had heard a voice saying that we needed to leave the house right now. We did leave the house and found a beautiful family that we taught.

"At the time I was envious that he got to hear a voice! Why wouldn't I get to have a miraculous experience when I was the one trying to be obedient? The lesson was that the Lord works through His stewardship channels--a senior companion in this case. And, importantly for me, that if we are doing the right thing at the right time and in the right way--doing our best--the Lord doesn't need dramatic and miraculous experiences to have us do his work. Rather, the peace and natural thoughts and desires lead us in righteous paths and enable us to be that conduit.

"I was serving a Spanish speaking mission in Northern Virginia and had started in the MTC during January of 1987. Our family had moved from Salt Lake to New York in June of that year, so no one from home was really keeping tabs on me. I was therefore not expecting much for Christmas or for my birthday, which was just before Christmas. Around Thanksgiving I got a check in the mail and a note from someone in our Salt Lake City ward. I decided to use the money for the people I was working with. I knelt down in prayer and told Heavenly Father how grateful I was for my blessings and that I was going to use that money and any more that came for others. It was a sacred and inspired moment. Well, checks started arriving right and left from people in Salt Lake and in New York, people I never even met, and it added up to over $1000 in no time. We did a secret Santa for a new member mother and her three children whom we had taught. She worked three jobs as a single parent. We paid the monthly rent for another family. We bought a bike to replace one that a missionary had lost. We did a lot of other things to help people out. Those who sent me gifts must have been prompted and inspired. Those who received gifts had prayers answered and greater testimony that God knew them personally and loved them deeply.

"I had been serving for over a year when I happened to read an account in the *Ensign* of a humble missionary in South America who heard the words 'Well done, thou good and faithful servant' at a point when he had wondered if his missionary service was successful. I hoped I could know the Lord was pleased with my service in such a clear way, but I never mentioned it to anyone. About nine months later when I had my exit interview with my mission president, he gave me a priesthood blessing and the words 'Well done, thou good and faithful servant' were included. I felt a strong spiritual witness that the Lord knew me and my heart and wanted to let me know that He was pleased."

**John Daniel Payne**

J.D. Payne served his mission in Rome, Italy. He enjoyed the Italian people for their vivacious personalities, willingness to engage with him, and their marvelous cultural history. Every day was an adventure filled with the whole spectrum of humanity from little children through adolescents, young adults, and older people. He watched the whole human experience flash before his eyes. He would think, "I wonder who I will meet today?" Sometimes people did not reciprocate his cheerful attitude. They could be mean, like the man who met them at the door with a gun or the one who kicked him in the shins when he tried to say hello. Whenever anyone responded negatively, Elder Payne would turn it over to the Lord and ask Him to flip it, to turn the negative into positive. Then he would give positive energy equal to what he had received as negative energy to the next person he met.

**Palmer Dickson**

Elder Palmer Dickson served his mission in the Mexico, Tampico Mission. He relayed the following story: "We needed to get to a meeting at 9 o'clock. We usually left our house at 8 to get to the meeting because we had to take a taxi, then a lancha (motorboat), then walk, then catch a bus, and then walk again. So we got outside at 8:15. That meant we could still make it easily on time but we wouldn't really get there early, unless everything worked out really well. As we waited on the side of the road for the taxi, several passed, but they were all full. It was now 8:30. I was starting to get antsy. I said a silent little prayer that we could find a taxi. After saying the prayer, we started walking to go to a place where there would surely be one. Probably in that same instant, a taxi came.

"The lanchas only leave once they are full. Some hold twenty passengers and some hold twenty-two. They are not allowed to take more. In the taxi I was still antsy about getting to the meeting on time. I remembered what President Call had taught us about having faith and not doubting (Mormon 9: 21, 25-27). I began to believe that it would be possible that we could be the 21st and the 22nd passengers on the lancha so that we could leave quickly. I silently prayed to Heavenly Father that He could grant me this tiny little miracle. I made sure to let Him know that I didn't want this miracle to give me knowledge that He lives. Instead, I let Him know that I believed that He could do it, and that I wouldn't doubt. I had had problems earlier in the week with doubting--our investigators were just not progressing. I had become discouraged.

"But I acted differently in the taxi. We were rounding the bend toward the lanchas. I could see the lancha, but it was far away. I could not see how many people were on it. Instead of peeking around to see how many were there, I stopped looking and just gave thanks to God and said, "I know that it's full except for two missionaries!"

"We got there. I saw the lancha super-full. I almost doubted, but I gave thanks again and said, 'Nope! No, no, no, we will be getting on that lancha.' I saw the man yank the engine starter of the little boat. Again I almost doubted, because whenever the engine starts it means that they are already leaving. But I said to myself, 'You are a God of miracles; I have faith that we can get on that boat.'

"The boat didn't move. We hurriedly got out, and the captain held up two fingers, which meant that only two people could get on. We were the only ones around, and we got on the boat. When he had held up the two fingers, I said to myself, 'Oooooooooh my goodness. It's all true. Everything is true. I knew Thou could do it!'

"The whole ride I was grinning. I was stunned. It was just so obvious that that had all happened because of a God who knows and cares for each and every single one of His billions of children. I feel happiness every time that I think about that experience."

**Eliza Dickson Wheeler**

"I served my mission in the Mar Vista, California area. Our mission president asked us to focus on families. We prayed and fasted to find a family to teach. We found pamphlets for houses for sale in our area and went to those houses, thinking that a family may have just moved in and was looking for a church to join. That was one point on my mission when I felt I was totally and completely lost in the work. I would go to sleep envisioning myself teaching a family. It was all I ever thought about--in the shower, in the car, while we were tracting--finding families. I was sure Heavenly Father would lead us to a family to teach and baptize.

"We did find a family to teach, but after five lessons, they told us not to come over anymore. What just happened? Weren't they supposed to be the miracle family that got baptized?

"We were teaching another family at that same time. They were members of the Spanish ward but not active. At that time only the husband, Adan Olivares, would listen to us. His wife, Dina, was more interested in Spanish soap operas. They had a seven year old daughter, Kimberly, and they invited us to her first communion party. Dina and Kimberly were still strongly Catholic, even though Dina had been baptized about ten years previously. Adan continued to invite us back, but Dina was quite cold to us. Adan started coming to church by himself, riding the bus. We learned that Dina had been baptized without fully understanding the commitment she was making. She wore pants to church, and a member told her she was not allowed inside because she needed to wear a skirt. That was the beginning of her inactivity.

"Adan had a side job selling food that he made. He had previously worked in a restaurant and learned how to cook well. He always sold his food on Sunday mornings. He said he needed the money, and if he came to church he would not make any money that week. We asked him to pray about it. He called us and told us with great excitement that he had an idea come to his mind that he had never thought of before. He would simply tell his clients to come to the house on Sunday evening to pick up their food instead of Sunday morning. Before this never seemed like an option because he thought he would lose all of his clients. He said all his clients were fine with the change. We explained that his idea came from the Holy Ghost. Heavenly Father was providing a way for Adan to continue his side job and still come to church. I left the area knowing that Adan was on his way to activity in the church, but didn't think that Dina or Kimberly would ever join him.

"A while later as I was working in the Visitors' Center, Dina Olivares rushed up to me and said, "Hermana Dickson!" She gave me a huge hug. I was shocked. This was not the Dina that I knew! Something happened after I left the area, and Dina had a change of heart. She and Kimberly had started going to church with Adan, and they loved it. She was so grateful to me for coming to teach them. I thought she never listened when I was teaching. In the following months, the Olivares family often came to the Visitors' Center and always sought me out. I learned that their relationship greatly improved. They had been close to separating months earlier. They were fully involved in the ward and were preparing to have Kimberly baptized. They decided to wait until Adan was ordained a priest so that he could baptize her.

"After I came home from my mission I learned that Adan and Dina were preparing to receive their temple ordinances. Dina asked me to be her escort as she received her endowment. It was a beautiful day to be in the temple with this family as they were sealed together. Adan is now the Elder's Quorum President in the ward.

"It was only after my mission that I realized that the Olivares family was the miracle family that Heavenly Father gave us.

"The blessings of a mission do not end once the mission is over. Whenever I have to prepare a lesson or talk about the Atonement, I think about how my mission gave me a greater understanding of the Atonement--of who Jesus Christ is, how he feels about me, and how he feels about everyone else in this world. We are nothing without him. Without a Savior, death and suffering are miserable. With the Savior, there is hope of a better world without suffering, there is hope for justification, there is hope that all wrongs will be made right, and there is hope in a resurrection. We will live with loved ones again."

**Vance Mellen**

"I had a terrible companion in the MTC. I'll call him Elder Smith. It was General Conference weekend when he snuck out with some other elders to go to a party with some girls. He was gone until the wee hours of the morning. The leader of the MTC was sitting in General Conference when the thought came to him, "Where is Elder Smith?" He left the conference and returned to the MTC, where he had an announcement go over the loudspeaker asking for Elders Smith and Mellen to come to the office. I went by myself in great trepidation and confessed that I didn't know where my companion was. I was told that we would both be sent home because it was my responsibility to watch over my companion. I explained that I had not known what to do, but that I had tried to stop him. When he eventually returned, he was sent home, but I was allowed to stay. He was the first of many difficult companions I worked with. My bishop had told me to love and serve companions that were hard. I decided to add a sense of humor and friendship to that list, and that served me well.

"I work hard to have spiritual experiences as part of my life now, and every now and again I will have one. The difference between these spiritual experiences and the ones I had on my mission are in frequency and intensity. The mission was like a spiritual life on steroids or spiritual downers on crack. The mission was one thousand times more intense than what a person will feel during normal spiritual experiences. I am lucky to have a spiritual experience once a week in my current life, but I had them far more intensely every single day, often ten times a day or more. I might go from giving a newly baptized convert the Holy Ghost and then only half an hour later tract into a self-proclaimed "Satan worshipping druid" on Christmas night (true story).

"Despite being with a companion that might be great or miserable, I often felt very lonely and unable to connect. There were many times when I wanted to love an investigator that I was teaching, but deep down inside, I could hardly stand them. Maybe they were lazy or just seemed too much of a "loser" to make it into the Church. I had to constantly battle against such judgmental and impatient thoughts.

"Little by little, over the first year of my mission I learned to feel and follow the Spirit. Most of my spiritual experiences were measured and small accomplishments wherein I learned what the Spirit really was, and what it was trying to tell me. These quiet kind of spiritual experiences, the daily grind, were the most valuable to me. This is how I learned the most.

"I also learned from bad experiences: bad companions, bad missionaries, unwilling members, lousy investigators, lack of support from ward mission leaders--all of these bad experiences humbled me and forced me to pray and build a friendship with Christ, who surely went through much of the same in His ministry. I learned patience. I learned to love and support even the most troublesome people. I learned to work things out; I learned when to call the mission president and when to put my foot down. Through these highs and lows on a mission I was whipped back and forth like a sapling in a Kansas tornado."

**Chadwick Mellen**

Elder Mellen was almost fourteen months into his mission in Leipzig, Germany, when he received word that his father had died. His journal record said:

"I received the worst news of my life. My district leader answered the phone early in the morning on a day I was preparing to transfer to a new city. He began to cry immediately and then handed the phone to me. President Moss called to inform me that my father died. My heart was so broken that I began to cry and tremble. Elder Szymonski asked me if I wanted a blessing, and I concurred. As soon as he put his hands on my head, he began to weep again. He assured me that my family was OK and that my Heavenly Father still loved me...I am now going to stay for a couple of days at the mission office in Leipzig.

"I've spent a great deal of time talking with President Moss. I know that I'm needed in this mission, but I almost want to ignore the promptings. [President Uchtdorf, the area authority at that time, told his mission president that Elder Mellen could go home for the funeral, but that if he did he would have to finish his mission in America.] This will be the hardest thing I will ever do. I'm not sure about trying to start over with a new city and a new companion. I'm not sure if I will be able to do much of anything. How am I going to get through this mess? I love my father so much. I also love and miss my family. My prayers are with them twenty-four hours a day. Heaven knows I'm going to need their prayers to accomplish the task at hand."

Elder Mellen's mother recorded these memories: President Moss was the mission president, and he called Elder Mellen early in the morning on a transfer day to tell him of the death of his father from a sudden and unexpected heart attack. President Moss had spoken to the area president at that time, Elder Uchtdorf, and relayed to me that he had encouraged him to stay on his mission in Germany. President Moss told Elder Mellen that he should pray about whether to leave Germany and go home for his father's funeral. After much prayer Elder Mellen, who really wanted to go to his father's funeral, decided to stay on his mission.

President Moss made arrangements for Elder Mellen to go into the mission home for a week to have some time to rest and process his great loss. He was treated so kindly. Hot meals, lots of sleep, and watching the video of his father's funeral helped to get him through a very hard time.

Elder Mellen's mother described her feelings at the end of her son's mission: "Chad had a request at the end of his mission, that I (who had never been out of the United States) would come to pick him up. He said that the image of returning home, embracing his father, and showing him that he was a changed person often got him through his difficult mission. He really couldn't face coming home alone. I flew to Frankfort, Germany, took a cab to the train station, found the train to Leipzig, rented a car, drove to the mission home, and found my son.

"The mission president had a final meeting for the eight missionaries going home. They sat in a circle and each missionary bore his testimony. When it came time for my son to bear his testimony, a bright light filled the room. I felt my husband's hands on my shoulders, and my son had a bright light like a fire around him. I knew then how special he really was, and that the light would always be with him. I knew that his earthly father would join with his Heavenly Father to protect and look after him. He left home as a boy and returned as a man, strong forever in his belief in the gospel and in Jesus Christ."

Chad Mellen reflected on his decision sixteen years later and wrote: "To this day I know I made the right decision to stay on my mission. I know the decision reflects the man I am today and how important commitments are to me. I'm not sure if I was the most effective missionary after that point and often felt bad for my companions. But I continued to try to serve the German people, whom I loved with all my heart, to the best of my ability. I taught and baptized a man from Africa and felt I was placed in that mission to bring him the gospel. I am uncertain if anyone else would have had that ability.

"I later learned that the entire mission had prayed and fasted for me. The people of Germany were so much kinder to me after my father died. I never again was yelled at as I knocked on numerous doors or approached people on the cobble stone streets of Germany.

I felt strongly that I had a large angel guarding and protecting me from that point on. I like to think that this was my father. It was an extremely difficult mission for numerous reasons. However, the one thing I will always be grateful for is that my mission helped convert me, and I gained a true testimony of the gospel of Jesus Christ."

**Matt Schults**

Elder Matt Schults was sent to Switzerland where he served for six months. He was transferred to Germany and thus had to apply to their government for permission to stay there. This was usually a routine matter, but this time the mission office lost his papers, something that had never happened before. He was six days overdue, and in spite of lawyers' efforts, his papers were stamped "Deported." He had to leave early the next morning. He spent the night packing and got to the airport at four AM. He felt extremely calm with the sense that this was what he was supposed to do. It helped that the situation had been presented to the first presidency of the Church, and they had responded that Elder Schults needed to return to the United States.

It was a long series of flights to Wisconsin where he would finish the last year of his mission. He hit a low point at two AM that night. He had been up for thirty-six hours and was exhausted. He went to the bathroom at the back of the plane, passing the empty stewardess chair. When he emerged a few moments later, a man was sitting in the chair reading. He looked up and asked, "Are you coming or going?" Elder Schults looked confused, and the man went on, "From your mission? You are going to Wisconsin. The Lord needs you there, and because you are obedient, you will find your purpose there." The man arose and walked to the front of the plane, and it was the last that Elder Schults saw of him. His words were comforting at that low point of exhaustion and doubt.

Elder Schults had been in Wisconsin for four months and was placed in a leadership position that involved zone conference training. After completing a conference about four hours from their home in Milwaukee, he and his companion were loading the van for the long trip back. He felt prompted to go to the bathroom, but he didn't have to go. Again came the prompting, and he ignored it. He then had a *very* strong impression to go to the bathroom, and so he went back into the church and found the bathroom.

When he entered, he found a missionary curled up in the fetal position, sobbing. Elder Schults lifted him up, put his arm around him, and began to comfort him. The missionary cried, "It's too hard. I can't do it." They went to a room and Elder Schults set up two chairs so they sat face to face, knees almost touching. The missionary continued to sob, pouring out his anxiety and discouragement. He then lifted his head and looked at Elder Schults for the first time. He glanced heavenward and began to laugh and then to cry again. Elder Schults was perplexed. The missionary cried out, "It was you!" "What do you mean?" asked Elder Schults.

The missionary revealed that he had been called to serve the Mong (Southeast Asian) population in Wisconsin. It was a tonal language, very difficult, and he was told that it would take him about eighteen months to learn it. During his thirteen weeks in the MTC, his anxiety became very severe, and he developed panic attacks stemming from his fear that he would not be able to learn the language. He decided on his last day in the MTC that he would go home. That night he had a dream. He was in Wisconsin and had been on his mission for a while. In the dream he was very discouraged and felt he should go home. A young man came, put his arm around him, and comforted him. The boy had a prosthetic eye with a pupil that did not dilate or constrict. It was the same eye that he saw when he lifted his head to look into Elder Schults' prosthetic eye. The missionary began to laugh, he said, "Because God knows me and loves me." He stayed on his mission, became proficient in the language, and went on to train others and be a very successful missionary.

Matt Schults said that his parents divorced when he was thirteen, and in the midst of this pain he became inactive for five or six years. He put his spiritual life in order and was able to come on a mission. He served a full two years and has been home for three years. Of the group of friends that left for their missions at the same time that he did, some stayed and some went home. He commented that he could see a huge difference between the two groups. The group who came home early lacked confidence and were beset with guilt that they had let down their families, while those who completed their missions were thriving.

In thinking about these stories, there are themes that shed light on how these missionaries successfully completed their missions. As I listened to their stories it occurred to me that all these missionaries described experiences that were difficult and stressful. They had to jump into a new language or they had callings that felt overwhelming or they dealt with exceedingly difficult companions or they had challenging investigators. In spite of these difficulties, they did not become depressed or overwhelmingly anxious, and they were able to remain on their missions.

There is a concept in psychiatry called resilience. It means that, given an experience of suffering, some develop a psychiatric illness while others do not. For example, not everyone who experienced 9/11 in New York City and Washington, DC, developed post traumatic stress disorder. Resilience is a complicated concept composed of many elements: genetics, epigenetic events which preceded the trauma (events that trigger genes to turn on or off), coping mechanisms learned from previous challenges, social support networks, and religious beliefs that offer a context of faith and hope. All are involved in resilience. So given equally stressful circumstances, some missionaries devolve into depression while others do not.

For those missionaries who are more resilient, there are other factors that contribute to their success. Obedience is the foundation of spiritual development. Vance Mellen advised my son before he went on his mission to be obedient, and all else would fall into place. When we are obedient, we can ask for blessings with faith that we will receive them. The Holy Ghost is more comfortable abiding in us if we are obedient.

I taught the Gospel Doctrine class for nine years, and often posed widely different questions that brought the same answer: pray and read the scriptures. There is good reason for this. These two activities connect us to Father in Heaven, Jesus Christ, and the Holy Ghost on a daily basis. When we read the scriptures regularly, we internalize them, and they guide us in times of difficulty. Missionaries have the great privilege of structured time each morning to read the scriptures. The rest of us have to consciously build it into our day.

As I consider these activities that lead to the growth of missionaries, I am reminded of an idea my husband shared with me. He is also a psychiatrist and is very interested in genomics. Genes are fascinating. We have them, but they can lie dormant for our whole lives if we don't activate them. For example, genes for cardiac and central nervous system well being can be activated by half an hour of aerobic exercise per day. Conversely, genes for diabetes can be activated by excessive daily sugar intake. My husband wondered if we have a set of Christ-like genes that can be activated by spiritual behaviors. These would include prayer, scripture study, acts of service, church and Temple attendance, and fulfilling one's callings. Maybe this increasing identification with the Savior explains the beauty of countenance one sees in those who have devoted their lives to the Gospel. I think missions accelerate this process because the whole day is set in a spiritual framework and expressed in the very behaviors I have mentioned.

Prayer, in particular, is one of the ways missionaries grow the most. Prayer is a two way street when it comes to communicating with the Lord. Most of the missionaries I have quoted described the vital importance of prayer on their missions. They indicated that prayer helped them rely on Heavenly Father, develop a friendship with Jesus Christ, and recognize the feeling of the Holy Ghost. My son, JD Payne, relayed an experience he had on his mission just before his first Christmas away from home. He received three letters in one week. The first was from his sister telling him she had a dreadful experience when she was endowed. The second was from his father telling him that he was very sick and afraid he might die. The third was from his girlfriend telling him she had been sexually assaulted. He called his mission president frantically and requested permission to call each of these dear people to comfort them. The mission president told him it was time for him to learn what prayer was all about. My son poured out his heart in prayer and received an overwhelming assurance that the Lord was there. His Father in Heaven provided a powerful sense of love and comfort. He felt the Lord saying, “I love you, and I’ve got this.” This experience became an anchor for him, and he could talk about prayer in a real way ever since.

Sometimes life feels like an endurance contest, but another message from these stories is that life is filled with light when we are serving others. Once a person catches the vision of service, the soul feels empty without it. If we have run out of people to serve, it is time to pray for more opportunities. There were times when I would go downstairs to the waiting room to find the elders in blue jeans and T-shirts. They had come from serving someone, usually an old lady. They would laugh happily as they described their back-breaking yard work (like clearing a back fence of nasty briar bushes), often performed under a hot and humid Virginia sun.

The ultimate goal of a mission is to develop the ability to love others. This greater ability to love comes by way of sacrifice. Parents who set aside their own needs to nurture a child understand that our love for our children grows as we sacrifice for them. A missionary is making many sacrifices just to be on a mission, and that is the beginning of the love he or she develops for others. As the spirit of a missionary is transformed, purified, and uplifted by his or her mission, he or she becomes more like the Savior. The following quotations from *The Infinite Atonement*, by Tad Callister[xx] capture this quality in both Jesus Christ and Heavenly Father:

"If sacrifice for others is the highest manifestation of love, then the Atonement of Jesus Christ is the grandest demonstration of love this world has ever known. The compelling, driving force behind his sacrifice was love, not duty or glory or honor or any other temporal reward. It was love in its purest, deepest, most enduring sense.

"From the premortal council until he breathed his last breath on Calvary, the Savior was impelled by unfeigned love, for 'in his love, and in his pity, he redeemed them' (D & C 133:53). Nephi was given an understanding of the abuse that would be heaped upon the Savior by an insensitive and ungrateful world: 'They scourge him, and he suffereth it; and they smite him, and he suffereth it. Yea, they spit upon him, and he suffereth it' (1 Nephi 19:9). Why such submission? Nephi gives the simple but profound answer: 'Because of his loving kindness and his longsuffering towards the children of men' (1 Nephi 19:9)."

Love is at the heart of the Gospel. Missionaries are fortunate to have that special time in life set aside to help them to develop love.

**Chapter 10: The Polar Express**

*On Christmas morning my little sister Sarah and I opened our presents. When it looked as if everything had been unwrapped, Sarah found one last small box behind the tree. It had my name on it. Inside was the silver bell! There was a note: "Found this on the seat of my sleigh. Fix that hole in your pocket." Signed, "Mr. C."*

*I shook the bell. It made the most beautiful sound my sister and I had ever heard. But my mother said, "Oh, that's too bad." "Yes," said my father, "it's broken." When I'd shaken the bell, my parents had not heard a sound.*

--"The Polar Express" by Chris Van Allsburg

The following story is a firsthand account by Matt Schults. I thought it deserved its own chapter:

Today is December 3, 2013. Exactly five years ago today I entered the MTC. My mission changed me. Through it I came to better know myself, and more importantly, my Savior. Every good thing that has come into my life since my mission is a result of my decision to serve.

Although much has changed since that unforgettable day, when a young 20-year-old boy said goodbye to his family for two years, not a day goes by that I don't reflect on my mission experience. I carry the faces of those I taught, the places where I served, and the sacred moments where God revealed Himself to me in my heart. Of all my experiences there may be none more sacred and revealing of God's love than the one involving the MTC, a home sick missionary, and a book, *The Polar Express*.

The day before entering the MTC, my bishop pulled me aside and said, "Matt, tomorrow, when you go to the MTC, everyone there is going to feel lost and alone. Make them feel at home." That advice resonated with me.

As the MTC Mission President concluded his speech and directed the parents out one door and missionaries out another I began to grasp what he meant. Tired, scared, lost, and alone I said goodbye, while desperately trying to hold on to my final exchanges with those I loved. I exited the building, grabbed my bags and walked to my apartment that I would call home for the next nine weeks.

With a heavy heart and teary eyes I found my way. There were four missionaries, two companionships, in each room. I was the last of the four to arrive. As I entered the room my attention was instantly drawn towards a missionary on the far side. He was sitting on the edge of his bed with his face buried in his hands. His name was Elder Newbold. He and Elder Pettingill were the neighboring companionship to Elder Talley and me.

Elder Newbold is small in stature and had I not known the missionary age requirement I would not have guessed he was nineteen years old. He was born and raised in Utah and comes from a large family. He is one of the most kind-hearted, humble, soft-spoken individuals I have ever met.

When I entered the room he glanced up from his defeated position with red puffy eyes and a runny nose, mustered up a halfhearted smile and returned to his hiding place. Initially, I assumed my attention was directed towards him because he looked as bad as I did, but I have since come to understand differently. It was he that I was to make feel at home.

One of the beauties of the MTC is that there is ample time for interaction amongst missionaries, especially with those within one's district. This made my job of befriending Elder Newbold that much easier. I made it a point to invite him to join in whatever activity I engaged in. However, I soon found out why he was hesitant to play basketball and why he stuck to Four Square. I had to abandon my initial plan and dream of us forming a Karl Malone and John Stockton MTC dynasty.

Although, basketball didn't suit us equally, we did find common ground. I saved him a seat next to me every day in the cafeteria. I made sure that our desks were next to each other in our classroom as well. During those marathon classroom days I would often tear off pieces of paper and send him little notes to break up the monotony and try to make him laugh. I would send notes asking him, "Do you think I'm cute? Check the box Yes or No." Or I'd comment on his outfit, "That tie really brings out the brown in your eyes."

Initially our conversation was brief and shallow. It could have been because his new roommate, whom he had never before met, was sending him secret loves notes asking if he thought he was cute. Nevertheless, our relationship grew and we became a source of comfort and friendship to each other.

Two and a half weeks into our nine-week stay we were beginning to get the hang of things. Suits and ties every day, a twenty-four/seven companion, and bedtimes were all becoming familiar. Unfortunately, there wasn't much we could do to prepare for our first Christmas away from home. It seemed that as soon as the initial shock was waning, the reality of Christmas away from home brought on another wave of homesickness.

Amidst the everyday hustle of MTC life there remained an underlying awareness of the coming Christmas without family. In the days leading up to Christmas, my mind was often caught up in what I could do to help make Christmas feel like home. The day before Christmas Eve, as I was praying before bed, the thought came to me of traditions. My family has numerous holiday traditions, each of which brings with it a host of joyful memories. In that moment I was filled with hope, a hope that if we could each incorporate one of our family's traditions we could save Christmas.

I excitedly arose from my knees and called all of my roommates into our room. As I began to make my proposal I could see a light of hope and excitement ignite in each of their eyes as well. Before I could even finish explaining my plan, Elder Pettingill and Elder Talley were both talking over each other recalling some of their favorite family traditions and the accompanying memories.

Elder Pettingill's most cherished tradition happened every Christmas Day. His family would bake Jesus a birthday cake and sing *Happy Birthday* to Him. The thought had never occurred to me to do such a thing and I didn't know how to get a hold of a cake. But I knew that the vending machine down the hall had hostess cupcakes and we could all sing. We could carry on the Pettingill tradition. His face beamed with excitement.

Elder Talley was next, his favorite tradition happened every Christmas Eve. He and his family would gather around the Christmas tree, often with a fire burning, and open just one gift. The rest were saved for Christmas Morning. He followed up his proposal with stories of gifts given and received and the laughs that always accompanied their tradition. Each of us had received a handful of gifts from parents and friends over the previous week. We could carry on the Talley tradition.

My tradition was simple and I knew we could manage it. Every Christmas Eve my family would gather in the living room and reflect on the events of the previous year. Then we would each take a turn and identify one thing for which we were most grateful. These were always some of my favorite conversations. The Spirit was always present and our love for each other and for Jesus Christ was never stronger. The spirit of gratitude is synonymous with Christmas and my heart was full with the anticipation of carrying on my tradition.

Amidst the excitement of realizing we would be able to

incorporate some of our favorite Christmas traditions Elder Newbold had faded into the background. As soon as I noticed his absence I looked towards his bed and found him in the exact spot I had three weeks earlier, sitting on the edge of his bed with his face in his hands. I called to him to ask for some of his Christmas traditions. He responded by staring at the ground and unconvincingly assuring us that our traditions would be good enough. Wanting him to feel the same excitement that we had uncovered, I persisted and assured him that we would do our best to pull off his favorite tradition

All of us sat quietly as Elder Newbold raised his head. Tears slowly filled his eyes and ran down his face as he told us of his favorite tradition, "Ever since I can remember, every Christmas Eve, after dinner, my family gathers around the fire place and my dad reads us *The Polar Express*. He always lets the youngest kids show the pictures and turn the pages. But five months ago my dad passed away and I will never be able to do that tradition again."

The room fell quiet as each of us internalized his situation. Would I have had the faith and courage to serve a mission if I were in his shoes? What could any of us say to comfort him? How could I possibly relate? My heart filled with compassion as I stared across the room at this great Elder. He truly had acted in faith and put God's will above his own.

In that moment the Spirit's voice whispered, "Check the present Melinda sent you." Melinda, my older sister, had sent me a Christmas package that I had received earlier that day. She had written me and asked if there was anything I needed. I had responded that I needed a scarf and a hat. Despite spending most of my life in Utah I had come ill-prepared for the cold.

The room remained still. Elder Newbold's tears had ceased. I gradually reached under the bed and pulled out Melinda's gift. The attention in the room shifted towards me. I slowly began unwrapping the large box. All eyes curiously followed my movements as I continued to pull away at the tape and strings that held it shut.

I opened the top of the rectangular box and reached in. As requested, I retrieved a scarf and then a hat. The bottom of the box was filled with candy and notes. I reached in the box a third time and pushed past the letters and sweets and felt something hard. My fingers traced the outline and found an edge. I pulled the rigid object to the surface and out of the box and in my hand was *The Polar Express!*

The Spirit filled the room. I was speechless. My eyes quickly shifted from the book in my hand to Elder Newbold. His eyes were fixed on the book and his face glowed. Tears began again to fill his eyes, only this time, a childlike smile came across his face. He then looked at me and said, "I know Christmas is going to be okay this year."

God's love was revealed to us and was encompassed in that simple phrase. God knows and loves each of us. We are his children. He loves us enough to send a homesick missionary a book. He loves us enough to let us know that we are never far from Him. He loves us enough to sacrifice his Son for us, that we may, one day, return to live with Him again.

The following day is one I won't soon forget. All four of us sat in a circle on the floor of our MTC apartment. The joy and love that filled our hearts was tangible, there was no other place we would have rather been. With gratitude in our hearts and smiles on our faces we carried on our Christmas traditions one by one. We each held a hostess cupcake in our hands as we cheerfully sang Happy Birthday to Jesus. We each took turns opening and showcasing one of the gifts we had received from our families. We reflected on the previous year and bore testimony of the Savior and expressed gratitude for the opportunity we had to bear His name and preach His gospel. And lastly, we each took our turn reading *The Polar Express* and showing each other the pictures.

This Christmas season there are surely those that are feeling lost and alone; make them feel at home. May we all be more mindful of those around us. Let us spare no effort this Christmas season letting those we love know of our love for them. Let us follow in the footsteps of our Savior and *succor the weak, lift up the hands which hang down, and strengthen the feeble knees.* Jesus was born of a virgin in a stable, He lived and loved perfectly, He was crucified for each one of us, and He arose from the tomb triumphant on the third day. Jesus Christ lives and because he lives we all have reason to rejoice this Christmas!

## Chapter 11: Reflections

*Batter my heart, three-person'd God, for you*
*As yet but knock, breathe, shine and seek to mend;*
*That I may rise and stand, o'erthrow me, and bend*
*Your force to break, burn, and make me new.*
*I, like an usurp'd town to another due,*
*Labor to admit you, but oh, to no end;*
*Reason, your viceroy in me, me should defend,*
*But is captiv'd, and proves weak or untrue.*
*Yet dearly I love you, and would be lov'd fain,*
*But am bethroth'd unto your enemy;*
*Divorce me, untie or break that knot again,*
*Take me to you, imprison me, for I,*
*Except you enthrall me, never shall be free,*
*Nor ever chaste, except you ravish me.*

--John Donne

Missionaries become strong as they are "whipped back and forth like a sapling in a Kansas tornado." My point in writing this book is that it is good for missionaries to stay through their whole mission so that they can have the maximum opportunity to grow spiritually. Going home early makes that growth slower and more difficult, but certainly not impossible. Spiritual growth is like the growth of a tree, which expands in concentric rings. As Elder Mellen expressed so well, "The mission was one thousand times more intense than what a person will feel during normal spiritual experiences, and spiritual experiences were much more frequent." That means the rings will be wider, and the tree will become stronger.

Most psychiatric conditions are treatable, and those who suffer with these problems can usually finish their missions. I know there are some circumstances which require intense treatment impossible to obtain while serving a mission. Sometimes it is necessary to relieve the stress of serving a mission before someone can recover, but these situations are uncommon in my experience.

I have spoken with several mission presidents and their wives to ask for their perspective on these issues. One commented that the ideal would be to keep every missionary until the end of his or her mission, but that as leaders, mission presidents and their wives have to consider the big picture. They have to worry about collateral damage to companions and even to wards. At what cost does a mission keep a missionary with psychiatric difficulties? We agreed that such decisions have to be made on a case by case basis after prayer and collaboration among all involved.

President Ed Scholz of the Munich, Germany mission said that it was one of his priorities to keep missionaries for the full time of their service. He sent home only three missionaries out of three hundred over his three years as a mission president. His goal was to keep them there and prepare them for leadership roles in the church after their return home. He also felt that it was important for them to stay because they had been through the temple and had made a commitment. With that came sacrifice. He had missionaries under his care whose parents got divorced or died, but they did not go home. President Scholz and his wife Lois helped them through it. He said that growth on a mission comes from converting oneself, from understanding the Gospel. A few of his missionaries left the Church after they returned home, but most remained faithful and strong. Some became outstanding Church leaders. He noted that the mission president's handbook said nothing about baptisms but rather talked about keeping the missionaries strong in the Church and preparing them for leadership.

Sister Scholz developed great skill in dealing with homesickness, a prevalent problem in this foreign mission with a difficult language and secular orientation.

The missionary would say, "I don't have a testimony anymore" rather than admitting, "I'm homesick." She told them they would have to wait a few weeks until someone arrived to replace them. In the meantime, they were to call her every day. They would talk for half an hour to an hour, and she would joke with them and make them laugh. After a week, they would forget to call. Then she would call them to see how they were doing, and usually this was enough after two weeks.

There were many other difficulties among the missionaries which the Scholz couple addressed in individual and creative ways, but Sister Scholz ended her comments by saying, "The most important thing for missionaries was to have a mission president who loved them."

A third mission president and his wife, Jack and Rosemary Wixom, were in charge of the Washington, DC, South mission. President Wixom commented that it was his priority to keep missionaries on their missions unless they became totally dysfunctional. He said most missionaries made significant spiritual progress. They blossomed at their own pace, aided by the discipline that a mission required. Many continued to flower after their missions, especially those elders who went home and married "cracker jack" women who ignited a spark in them. President Wixom added that Heavenly Father gives us many chances to grow.

President Wixom said that some missionaries never really got it--why they were there. It was not a mental health issue, but one of spiritual health. How well did they get the Spirit? For others the problem was narcissism. He said they failed to grow up on their missions. (Adolescents are normally narcissistic, but it is a state of mind that most of us outgrow. Those who don't go on to exhibit narcissistic personality disorder.) A very small percentage of his missionaries went home and became inactive.

Some of his missionaries revealed after their missions that they were homosexual. He said that the ones who have kept in touch with him are celibate and are still strong in the Church.

At the end of our discussion he added that he loves all his missionaries dearly.

A final mission president I spoke with was President Craig Pacini, who served as president of the Rome, Italy, mission. He believed in keeping missionaries on their missions if at all possible. He felt that even if a missionary had a legitimate reason for going home, if he did so he would always be left with a nagging feeling that he had let the Lord down. He felt that mission presidents should be grateful for every missionary, regardless of their weaknesses, because the Lord sent them where he did for good reasons.

His approach with his missionaries was to develop a relationship with them that allowed them to share their opinions with him and develop their leadership skills. He did not believe in being a leader who just handed down orders. He wanted his missionaries to feel confident and respected.

For example, President Pacini said that when he assumed leadership in the mission, there were extremely rigid rules in place governing the relationship between elders and sisters. The rules had developed from problems with which the previous mission president had dealt. President Pacini decided to leave the rules in place for awhile, but after nine months he felt it would be good to relax them a bit. He called the zone leaders to discuss it, and they answered, "No, we are comfortable in our relationship with the sisters." So the rules remained.

As a second example, President Pacini said that he decided he did not want to have a teaching conference with new missionaries as soon as they arrived in Rome because they were too jet-lagged and stressed. He wanted to postpone this to their third month and then have another session at their one year mark. The zone leaders vetoed the one year conference but agreed with the three month one, so that is what they did. At that conference, he had the new missionaries fill in a plan based on their own feelings about what they wanted to accomplish on their missions. Each missionary kept a copy as a guideline for his or her own mission.

At this conference, he also had the missionaries make a list of all the qualities they felt a missionary should have. Each one then decided which qualities he would like to improve. They took the list to their leaders and asked for their help in developing these qualities.

President Pacini also carefully gathered information from the zone leaders before each transfer to make wise, informed decisions. If a transfer would derail the teaching of a certain investigator, it was not made. If it was important to separate a pair of missionaries, the transfer was made.

In all these examples, I could see that President Pacini strengthened his missionaries and conveyed deep respect for their free agency. He also told them that there was no such thing as a perfect missionary. They often saw qualities in other missionaries which they assembled into a "mythical missionary." In comparison with this myth, they became discouraged and felt that they should give up and go home. He told them that discouragement is from the devil, and if they wondered how they were doing, they should ask Father in Heaven. He called them, so He should know. President Pacini said to remember how close Heavenly Father was to missionaries and that He would support them.

He taught them to do their job as missionaries and then turn it over to the investigators. It was their responsibility to use their free agency to make a decision. Conversions, he added, are nonverbal; they are done through the Spirit.

He instructed his missionaries, "Don't look back after your mission with regrets because you see what you could have done differently. You have more mature eyes, and it is just the adversary trying to discourage you." In all his comments, I could hear his love for his missionaries and his efforts to protect them from self-doubt and blame. He told them that missionary service is not a program. It is an opportunity to exercise deep faith. Under his good care, baptisms increased by 144%. This brought great hope to the struggling Italian members. He told the missionaries that if they worked hard, Rome would be the site of a new temple-- and that is indeed now happening.

The potential for spiritual growth in missionaries is immense. It is evident in the missionaries' stories in this book how much Heavenly Father and Jesus Christ love them and how personal and detailed this love is. Their growth is expressed in their increased reliance on Heavenly Father. It is there in the friendship developed with the Savior. It is present in the increased sensitivity to the Holy Ghost. They become more disciplined and humble through their obedience. They learn to rely on prayer and the scriptures, and as they become stronger in these areas they develop greater faith, patience, and hope. They learn that enduring to the end brings peace and joy. They learn to love others, even those who initially didn't seem very lovable. However, to obtain these blessings, to become strong, they need to try difficult things.

I did not serve a mission, though several kind missionaries told me my work with them *was* my mission, but I chose to do something difficult in being a psychiatrist for forty years. Many patients were not easy to treat. I've written a poem about one patient with borderline personality disorder which describes how it feels to tackle a hard case. This poem is based on the mythological visit of Thor and Loki (Norse gods) to the Giants. The Giants put them to several tests: one was to lift a cat (a symbol of the world spirit). Had Thor succeeded, the world would have ended, but in managing to lift one of her paws, Thor terrified the Giants.

*If you want to be strong, you have to lift something heavy.*
*Come on, then. I'll lift you.*
*You're little and light, but I feel your dark and heavy spirit.*
*Why are you on all fours?*
*Why is your back arched?*
*Why do you hiss and spit at me?*
*I can barely get two of your paws off the ground.*
*Try as I might, strain as I do,*
*Grappling with your surprising strength I am spent:*
*Strength born of bitterness, slow rage that has simmered for ages on a fire tended with meticulous care, fed with evidence of the world's cruelty.*
*You say you want to die, but you enjoy hurting too much to give it up.*
*Hurting yourself, hurting others--what is the difference?*
*Soon I will be covered with the long scars that your claws rake into me.*
*But my slow, steady lifting will continue. Week by week for twenty years.*
*I will push against your arched back until I have lifted you clean into the air,*
*Away from your suffering,*
*And the world will not end.*
*But I will be strong.*

This is not a pleasant poem, but I hope it conveys the difficulty of the work. My years as a psychiatrist refined me. I learned not to judge, to be patient, and to love those I sought to help. In choosing to do difficult things, we can become strong.

The following final missionary story encapsulates the difficulties of missions. Maria Dickson Rees writes about how a disappointing time in her mission eventually strengthened her spirituality:

"We arrived a bit late to fast and testimony meeting because as usual, we ran from investigator to investigator to pick them up for church. We had planned on ten being able to come. Well, none of the investigators came with us. So for the first little bit of the meeting, I looked around in hopes of seeing any of the others we had invited walk into the meeting. None of them came. Not one of the ten that had committed to coming actually came. The frustration I was feeling the whole morning grew into anger and the tears came. I thought about how I was sweating, uncomfortably hot, starving (from fasting), with a sore throat, and without one investigator present at church. Sitting there sweating and sobbing in front of everyone else made me feel even worse. And then I felt disappointed in myself for being disappointed. As I looked at the words of the hymns through my watery eyes, my thoughts turned to God. 'Heavenly Father, this is miserable. I'm hot and starving and none of our investigators came! Why didn't any of them come? Even after all of our hard work?' Then I tried to compose myself as members bore their testimonies, but I wasn't listening very well to what they were saying...until one of the young women got up. I don't know if she saw me crying or not, but she bore her testimony of the power of missionary work, and her words touched my spirit and answered my prayers. Then I started crying again because I was feeling Heavenly Father's love and mercy for me! I was strengthened by her testimony and by the Spirit, and I could compose myself. I realized that everything was going to be okay, despite all the thoughts I was having earlier."

After this experience, Sister Rees recalled these words of Elder Jeffrey Holland which she heard in the MTC in Sao Paulo, Brazil:

> "Anyone who does any kind of missionary work will have occasion to ask, Why is this so hard? Why doesn't it go

better? Why can't our success be more rapid? Why aren't there more people joining the Church? It is the truth. We believe in angels. We trust in miracles. Why don't people just flock to the font? Why isn't the only risk in missionary work that of pneumonia from being soaking wet all day and all night in the baptismal font?

"You will have occasion to ask those questions. I have thought about this a great deal. I offer this as my personal feeling. I am convinced that missionary work is not easy because salvation is not a cheap experience. Salvation never was easy. We are The Church of Jesus Christ, this is the truth, and He is our Great Eternal Head. How could we believe it would be easy for us when it was never, ever easy for Him? It seems to me that missionaries and mission leaders have to spend at least a few moments in Gethsemane. Missionaries and mission leaders have to take at least a step or two toward the summit of Calvary."

At the close of this book, I would like to include a spiritual experience of my own to add my voice to those of the missionaries who have shared so generously. I have had some wonderful spiritual experiences, but this one was the most powerful and most helpful. So that you will understand why it was helpful, I will share the fact that our father never told any of his five children that he loved us, nor did he show any interest in my inner life. As my parents aged, my mother encouraged him to tell us. His answer was classic Dad, "Margaret, words are cheap. If they don't know by now after all my hard work, they never will." He died without telling us, and since I value words so much, I was left doubting that he did love me.

One day I was on my knees praying. I must have been anxious or tired, but my prayer seemed to bounce off the ceiling and fall to the floor. I decided to pray visually, something I had never done before. I thought of Ezekiel 1: 26-28:

*And above the firmament that was over their heads was the likeness of a throne, as the appearance of a sapphire stone: and upon the likeness of the throne was the likeness as the appearance of a man above upon it.*

*And I saw as the colour of amber, as the appearance of fire round about within it, from the appearance of his loins even upward, and from the appearance of his loins even downward, I saw as it were the appearance of fire, and it had brightness round about.*

*As the appearance of the bow that is in the cloud in the day of rain, so was the appearance of the brightness round about. This was the appearance of the likeness of the glory of the Lord. And when I saw it, I fell upon my face, and I heard a voice of one that spake.*

As I envisioned the beautiful throne of God with its marvelous colors, it seemed to me that my spirit left my body. I went to Heaven and sat on the lap of my Heavenly Father. In this experience He folded me in His wings, soft and warm and filled with tenderness. He told me that he approved of my life. He radiated immense love beyond anything we have experienced on this earth.

The Book of Mormon says: "And no tongue can speak, neither can there be written by any man, neither can the hearts of men conceive so great and marvelous things as we both saw and heard Jesus speak; and no one can conceive of the joy which filled our souls at the time we heard him pray for us unto the Father" (3 Nephi 17:17). That is what this experience was like. His love filled me with joy and with a wish to be with Him forever. I looked to His side and saw my Heavenly Mother, and beyond her I saw my brother Jesus Christ. I was home with my heavenly family. I thought of the last verse of the song, "My Shepherd Will Supply my Need" by Isaac Watts[xxi]:

The sure provisions of my God
Attend me all my days;
O may thy house be mine abode
And all my work be praise:
There would I find a settled rest
While others go and come,
No more a stranger, nor a guest,
But like a child at home.

I had to return to my body, but as I did so the Holy Ghost came with me, and wrapping his arms around me, assured me that he would remain with me. This experience was exactly the one I needed. It has stayed with me all my life. I realized that my earthly father was limited in his ability to convey love, but I have another Father whose love is boundless and infinitely joyous.

In defense of my father, let me add that as the years have passed since his death, I have often thought about his answer to my mother, that his manner of conveying love was through action. I recently remembered that my parents visited us one August when my father was in his early eighties. He had grown up on a farm and continued to be a gardener all his life. He came out to our orchard to help me weed. He was too old to kneel down so he stretched out full length on his side to pull the weeds, laboriously getting up and moving with me from tree to tree. He was wearing his jungle helmet, issued to him in World War II when it looked like he was going to fight in North Africa.

It was a very hot and humid day, and as I look back on this experience I realize no one would ever have come out to weed with me unless he loved me. This experience occurred about twenty years after Heavenly Father had comforted me, but it was wonderful to realize that I have two loving fathers. Why does it take a lifetime to resolve these questions?

Growth is slow, but it is important to remember that Heavenly Father provides us with the experiences we need to help us move forward. Serving a mission is one such experience, one that young missionaries choose to do.

Whenever I think about the amazing experience I described as I was praying, I also think that I want everyone to have access to the love our Father feels for us. What a difference this would make in this angry, suffering, sad world. His love is a magnet that draws our souls to Heaven. Once one has tasted of this love, there is no more disposition to do evil, but to do good continually. Missionary work is the way this message is spread among His children. It is another reason that it is so important to support missionaries, to help them complete their missions. It is true that missionaries are "whipped back and forth like a sapling in a Kansas tornado," but these challenges do make them stronger in faith, patience, and love. I am sure that Father in Heaven and His Son especially love them for their willing sacrifice.

## Glossary

**Anoxia** – lack of oxygen

**Antidepressant** – medication to treat depression. Current medications include:

- **SSRI** (specific serotonin reuptake inhibitors) Ex: Prozac, Zoloft, Paxil, Celexa, Lexapro, Viibryd, and Brintellix (also a serotonin modulator)
- **SNRI** (serotonin norepinephrine reuptake inhibitor) Ex: Effexor, Pristiq, Cymbalta, and Fetzima
- **DS** (dopamine serotonin) Ex: Wellbutrin

**Character disorder** – a psychiatric diagnosis that implies the condition is chronic, describing a personality. People with this diagnosis often do not seek treatment themselves but are referred by family members or the Courts. Ex: borderline, narcissistic, or sociopathic personality disorders

**Cognitive behavioral therapy (CBT)** – a structured and formal approach to therapy in contrast to insight oriented therapy in which the patient talks about his problems in an unstructured way. CBT is very useful for obsessive-compulsive disorder, anxiety disorders, and depression.

**Cognitive impairment** – a problem with the thinking functions of the brain. Can be due to trauma, strokes, drug abuse, developmental conditions like Attention Deficit Hyperactivity Disorder, congenital problems, or the long term damage associated with mood disorders

**Comorbid** – several illnesses present at the same time

**Executive functioning** – carried out mostly by the frontal lobe of the brain to assist in performing the chores of life, including organization, initiation of tasks, working memory, reasoning, cognitive flexibility, problem solving, planning and execution of tasks, time management, and sustaining attention

**Frontal lobe** – the newest and most forward cortical area of the brain that is in charge of executive functioning

**Macroscopic** – large enough to perceive with the naked eye as opposed to microscopic

**Major tranquilizer** – a class of medications which modulates the dopamine receptor used to treat psychiatric disorders like schizophrenia and Type I bipolar disorders; also used for Type II bipolar disorder and severe obsessive compulsive disorders. Ex: Abilify, Seroquel, Zyprexa

**Mentalization** – the ability to understand mental states that underlie the behavior of oneself and others; a type of meditation to help people become more self-aware. Useful for conditions like borderline personality disorder.

**Mood stabilizers** – medications used to stabilize mood in bipolar patients and to calm aggression in people with strong tempers from any cause. Some of them also function as anticonvulsants in those with seizure disorders. Ex: Depakote, Lithium, Tegretol, Lamictal

**Morbidity** – illness

**Neuron** – one type of brain cell

**Neurotransmitters** – chemical messengers that communicate between neurons. There are at least one hundred and fifty of them in the central nervous system, but the following three are widespread and regulate many important neurological functions:

- **Serotonin** – regulates mood, appetite, and sleep. Contributes to memory and learning.
- **Norepinephrine** – regulates concentration, anxiety (fight or flight behavior), cognitive functions
- **Dopamine** – regulates alertness, concentration, reward motivated behavior, aggression, and muscle movement

**Neurotropic** – localized to nerve tissue

**Permeable** – able to allow substances to cross through barriers like the cell wall or the blood brain barrier

**Psychomotor** – agitated feelings and physical movements

## Bibliography

[i] Holland, Jeffrey R. "Like a Broken Vessel," *Ensign*. Salt Lake City, Utah: Church Magazines, November, 2013. p 40-42.

[ii] Jamison, Kay Redfield. *Exuberance*. New York: Random House, 2004. p 24.

[iii] American Psychiatric Association. *Diagnostic and Statistical Manual of Mental Disorders, Fifth Edition*. Arlington, Virginia: American Psychiatric Association, 2013. p 124.

[iv] Shakespeare, William. *Hamlet. The Complete Works of Shakespeare*. Garden City: Doubleday and Co., Inc., 1936. p748.

[v] American Psychiatric Association. *Diagnostic and Statistical Manual of Mental Disorders, Fifth Edition*. Arlington Virginia: American Psychiatric Association, 2013. p 160-161.

[vi] Styron, William. *Darkness Visible*. New York: Random House, 1990. p 46.

[vii] American Psychiatric Association. *Diagnostic and Statistical Manual of Mental Disorders, Fifth Edition*. Arlington, Virginia: American Psychiatric Association, 2013. p 222-225.

[viii] American Psychiatric Association. *Diagnostic and Statistical Manual of Mental Disorders, Fifth Edition*. Arlington, Virginia: American Psychiatric Association, 2013. p 208-209.

[ix] Allen, Woody. *Without Feathers*. New York: Random House, 1975.

---

[x] American Psychiatric Association. *Diagnostic and Statistical Manual of Mental Disorders, Fifth Edition*. Arlington, Virginia: American Psychiatric Association, 2013. p 237.

[xi] Hallowell, Ned, and Ratey, John. *Delivered from Distraction.* New York: Ballantine, 2005.

[xii] American Psychiatric Association. *Diagnostic and Statistical Manual of Mental Disorders, Fifth Edition.* Arlington, Virginia: American Psychiatric Association, 2013. p 59-61.

[xiii] Hopkins, Gerard Manley. "Pied Beauty." *Chief Modern Poets of England and America.* New York: The MacMillan Co., 1962. p 61-62.

[xiv] American Psychiatric Association. *Diagnostic and Statistical Manual of Mental Disorders, Fifth Edition.* Arlington, Virginia: American Psychiatric Association, 2013. p 242-243.

[xv] Robinson, John. *Look Me in the Eye.* New York: Random House, 2007. p. 20.

[xvi] Yeats, William Butler. "The Second Coming." *Chief Modern Poets of England and American.* New York: The MacMillan Co., 1962. p 125.

[xvii] American Psychiatric Association. *Diagnostic and Statistical Manual of Mental Disorders, Fifth Edition*. Arlington, Virginia: American Psychiatric Association, 2013. p 102.

[xviii] American Psychiatric Association. *Diagnostic and Statistical Manual of Mental Disorders, Fifth Edition.* Arlington, Virginia: American Psychiatric Association, 2013.

---

[xix] Groberg, John. *In the Eye of the Storm*. Salt Lake City: Bookcraft, 1993. p 114,117.

[xx] Callister, Tad. *The Infinite Atonement*. Salt Lake City, Utah: Deseret Book, 2000. p 158.

[xxi] Watts, Isaac. "My Shepherd Will Supply My Need." The Mormon Tabernacle Choir CD. Salt Lake City, Utah: Mormon Tabernacle Choir, 2003.

# ABOUT THE AUTHOR

L. Marlene Payne, M.D., has been a psychiatrist for forty years. She went to Northwestern University undergraduate and medical school in Chicago, Illinois, then did a one year internship in internal medicine at Northwestern University. She continued her training with a two year residency in adult psychiatry and a two year fellowship in child and adolescent psychiatry at Georgetown University in Washington, D.C. She was an Assistant Clinical Professor at Georgetown for twenty years, supervising child and adolescent psychiatry fellows. She practiced psychiatry in McLean, Virginia, for thirty-six years until her retirement in July, 2013. She received the highest award given by the American Psychiatric Association, the Distinguished Life Fellow of the American Psychiatric Association, for her years of service to the community. She is married to Dr. John Payne, also a psychiatrist, and they have three children and three grandchildren. She is currently a temple worker and compassionate service leader in Relief Society.

20052947R00085

Made in the USA
Middletown, DE
13 May 2015